NEIL GOLDBERG

OTHER PEOPLE'S PRESCRIPTIONS

ESOPUS BOOKS

Art that takes the form of documentation by the means of mechanical reproduction can have an affectless interface. The camera is a fly on life's wall, a reducer of the passing show to a catalog. Neil Goldberg's art is not that kind of art. Goldberg is a Romantic. He doesn't make art out of the ordinary and banal—that would be an easy mistake to make—because to a Romantic, nothing is ordinary or banal. Everything is amazing already—people's elbows, people's eyeglasses, people carrying shopping bags with groceries from Whole Foods.

It's true that there is a distinct "foundness" in Goldberg's art. That is the MO, and, in his sort of art (maybe in any sort of art), the MO is half the story. But his objets trouvés are human beings, and those happen to be the objets human beings understand the least. We can predict the behavior of a planet better than we can predict the behavior of the person sitting across from us at the breakfast table. And we certainly know more for sure about the planets than we do about the people standing next to us on the subway platform. The people on the platform are the subjects of Goldberg's visual art.

In many ways, New York City is all facade, a wall-to-wall storefront where you have no idea what is going on in the back of the shop. You suspect that maybe it's nothing very interesting, or even that maybe there is no back of the shop. But how would you know? They never let you in past the displays. You're always out on the sidewalk. Except for the subway. The subway is real. On the subway, everything is what it is. Even more than the jury pool or the DMV, the subway is where whatever ancestral, cultural, or class-positional baggage you bring to the occasion counts for nothing. There is no upstairs or backstage on the subway.

This inescapable egalitarianism of urban life is a key perception in Goldberg's work. He is interested in the way human beings in roughly the same circumstances react in roughly the same ways, but never in *exactly* the same ways. There is a pattern, a visual rhythm, in, say, the faces of subway riders who just missed their trains. ("There is a train directly behind this one," they tell us. Yes, of course there is. How could there not be one? This is a subway track. The question is, How *far* behind? They never say.)

In *Other People's Prescriptions*, the artist is interested in the variance within another common condition: wearing corrective lenses. Notice the care he takes to compose every shot the same: that's the rhythm. And at the center of each frame sits the mark of individuation: the prescription. "Walk a mile in my shoes." Yes, I might learn that your feet are bigger than mine. But "Walk a mile wearing my glasses"? That's where we are likely to appreciate how differently we are made.

Eyeglasses are a metaphor: they stand for perception. How do we know that the world I see is also the world that you see? Stanley Cavell had an answer: photography. A photograph (he was thinking about the cinema) is a representation by a mechanical apparatus that nevertheless looks like the world we humans see. If a machine can "see" what we see, and if we all recognize the photographic image as "real," then we're not trapped in a solipsistic dream.

But is that world we see in fact the world as it is? "Magnifying glasses are like a high heel to a short leg," wrote the 17th-century English philosopher Margaret Cavendish. She was skeptical: How could a device designed to distort things—by making them appear bigger or closer or in sharper focus—also make our perceptions of them truer? She thought that they could not, that we are fooling ourselves when we believe that a microscope gives us a more accurate image of a plant or a microorganism. It falsifies. It makes the thing bigger than it really is.

We have the same, though vaguer, since we are not philosophers, sense of unease when we look at these photographs. These people are not seeing the world, we think; they're seeing what looks to us like a distorted, compressed, miniaturized rendition of the world. As a lifetime glasses wearer (never cool enough for contacts), I know that with my glasses off things have a fullness, a warmth, a three-dimensionality, that I don't get while wearing them. Yet for all practical purposes, the world-in-a-lens is the world I know and deal with every day.

But in Goldberg's series, this thought—we change perceptions with prescriptions—is given another twist. His subjects are looking through lenses, but he is looking at his subjects through a lens—the camera lens. Looking at the photographs, we are seeing the image created by a lens on lenses.

And what are we looking with? Another lens. Eyeballs are the eyeglasses that evolution has given us. Yet without them, we would all be Mr. Magoo. The eye puts color where there is none, turns 24 frames a second into continuous motion. The eye is a liar, but it's our liar. It makes the world habitable for us. And that's all that natural selection requires. It does not require that we know the truth about the world, only that we know enough to cope with it. Which is what I think these witty, and in their way, joyous photographs are reminding us.

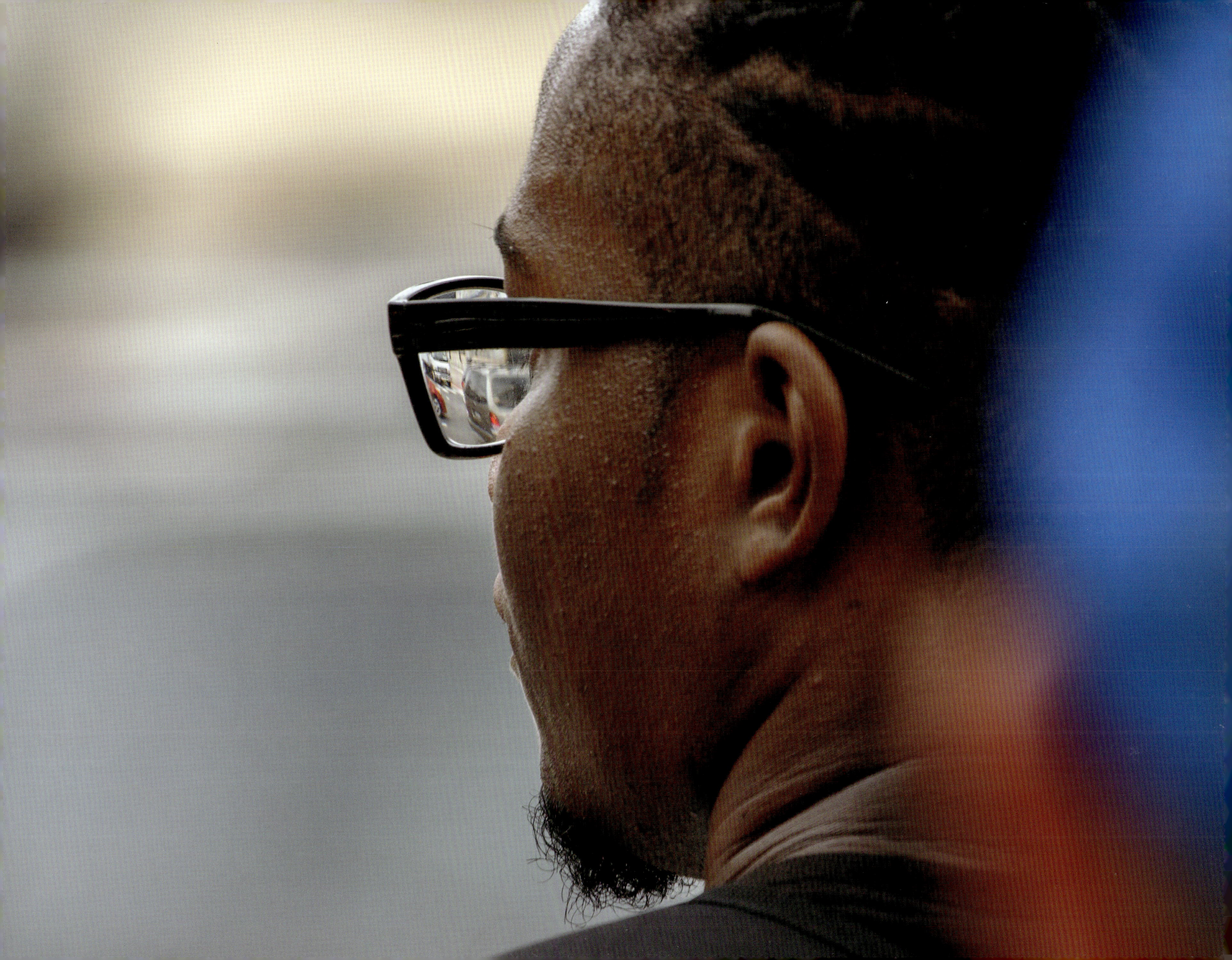

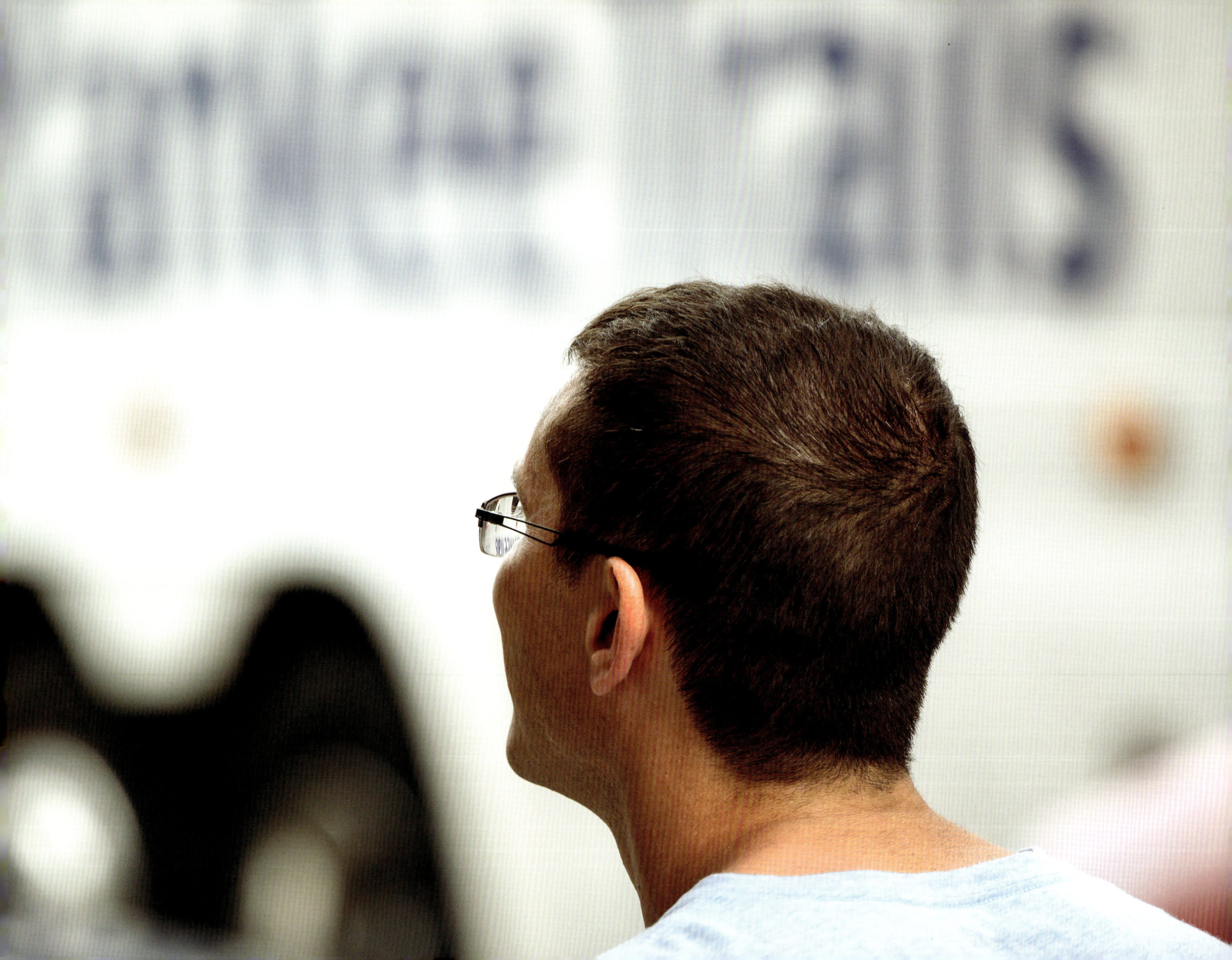

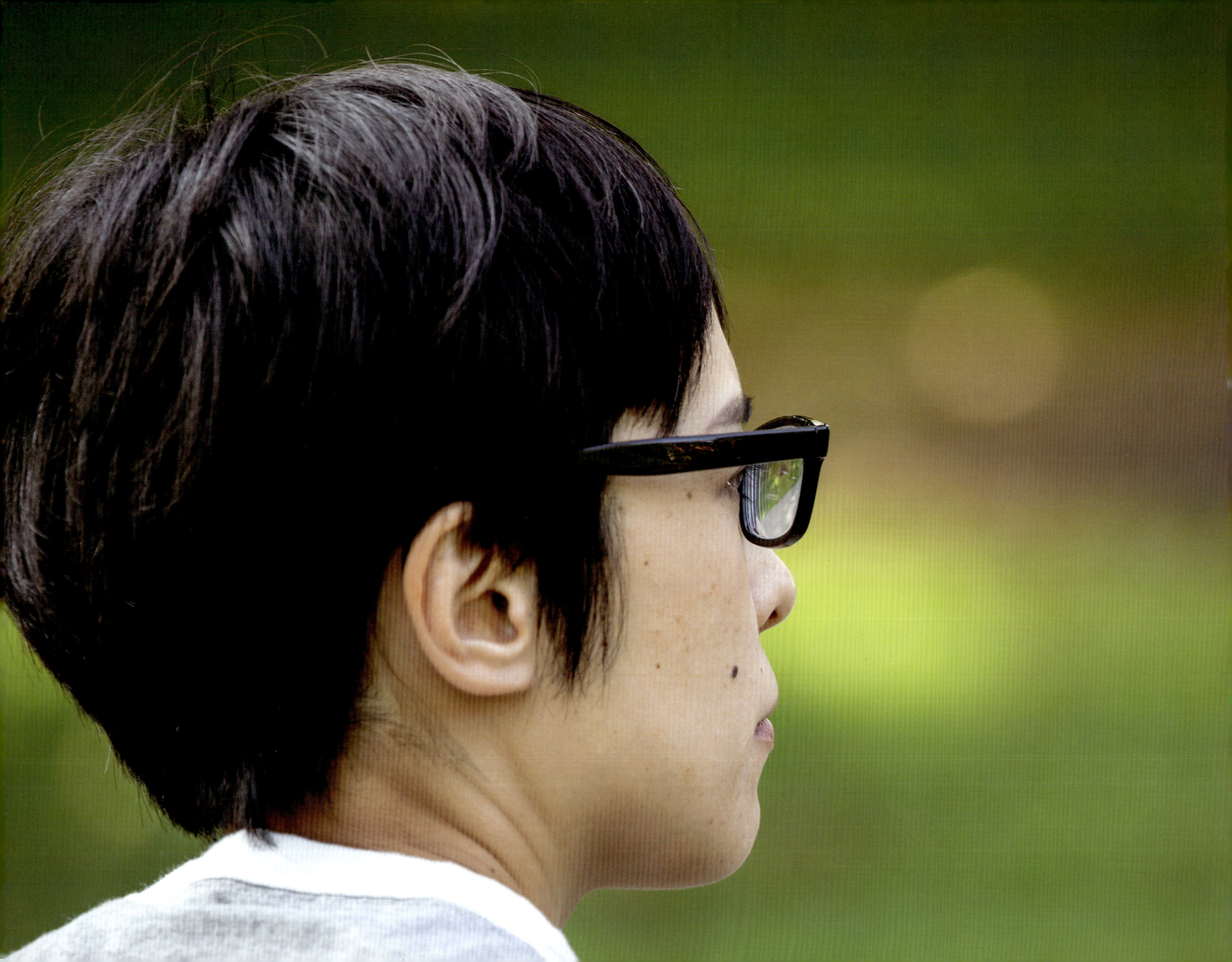

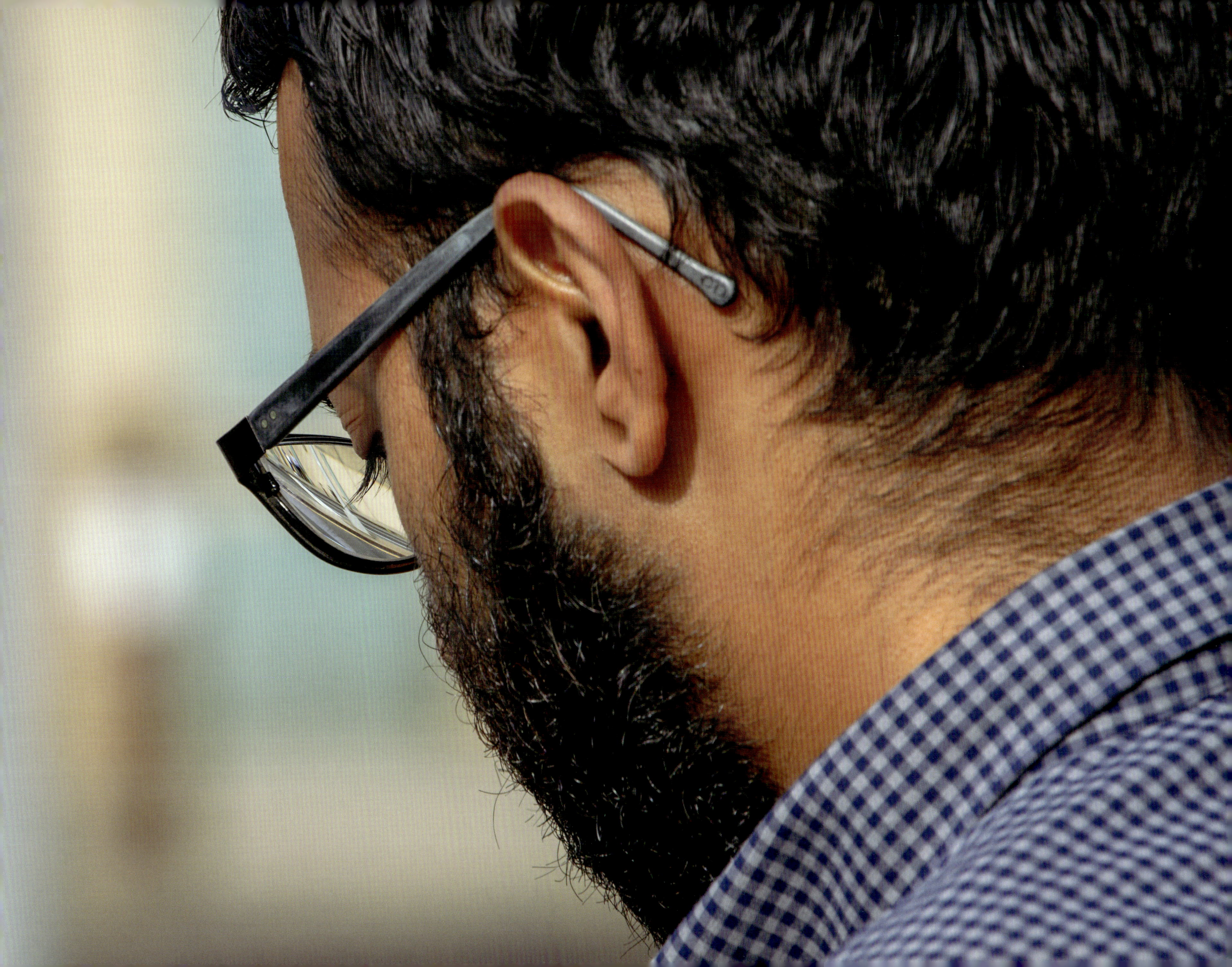

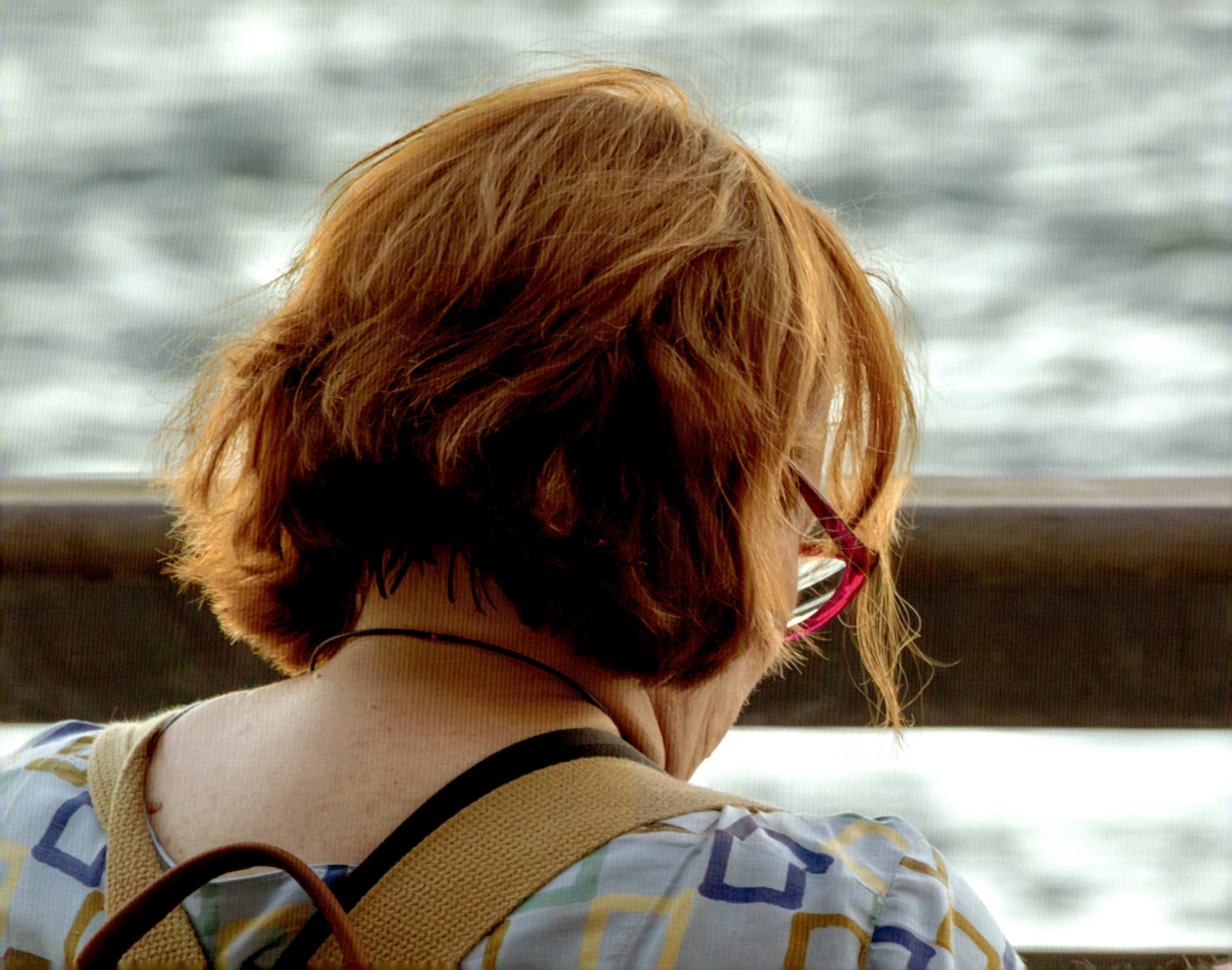

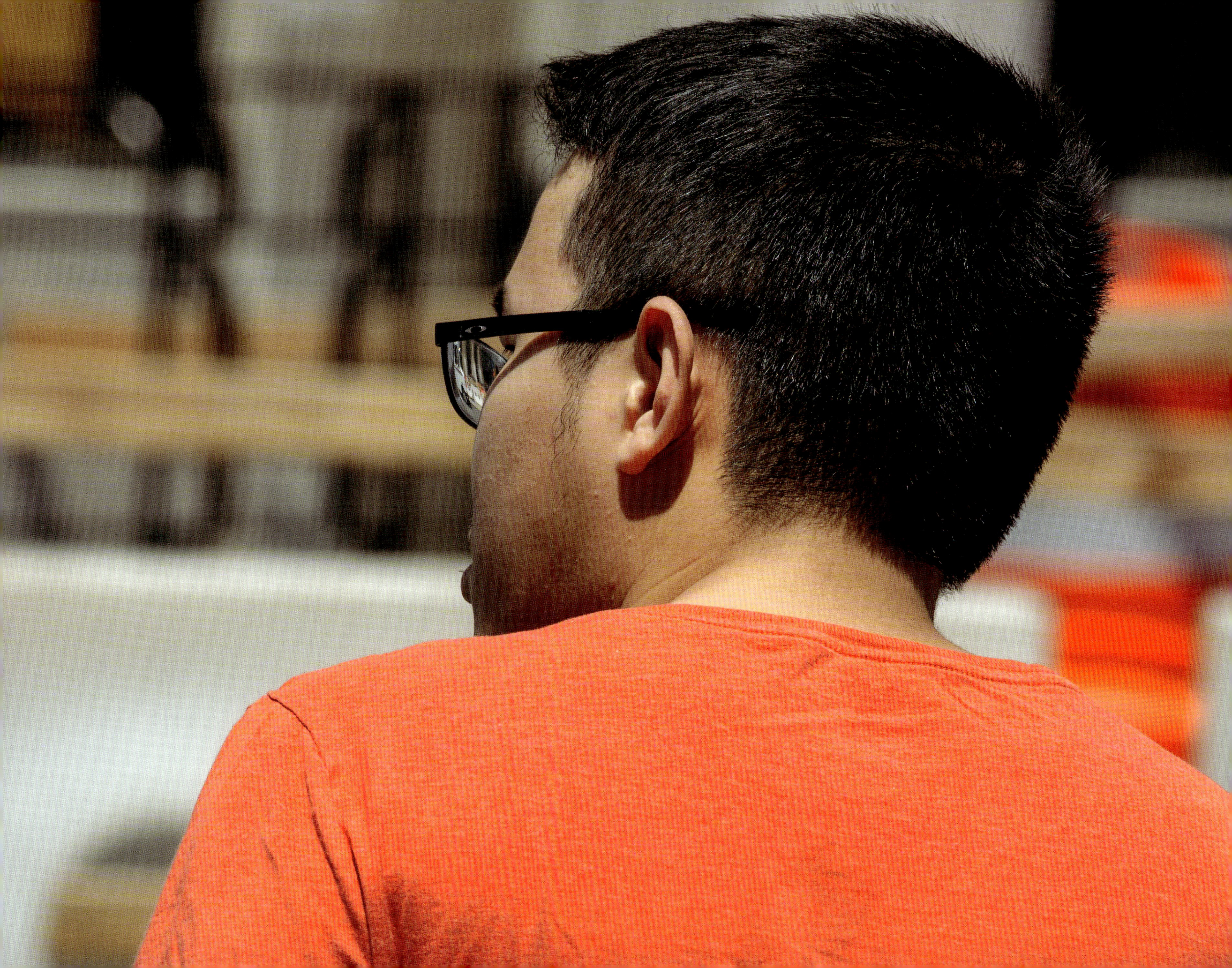

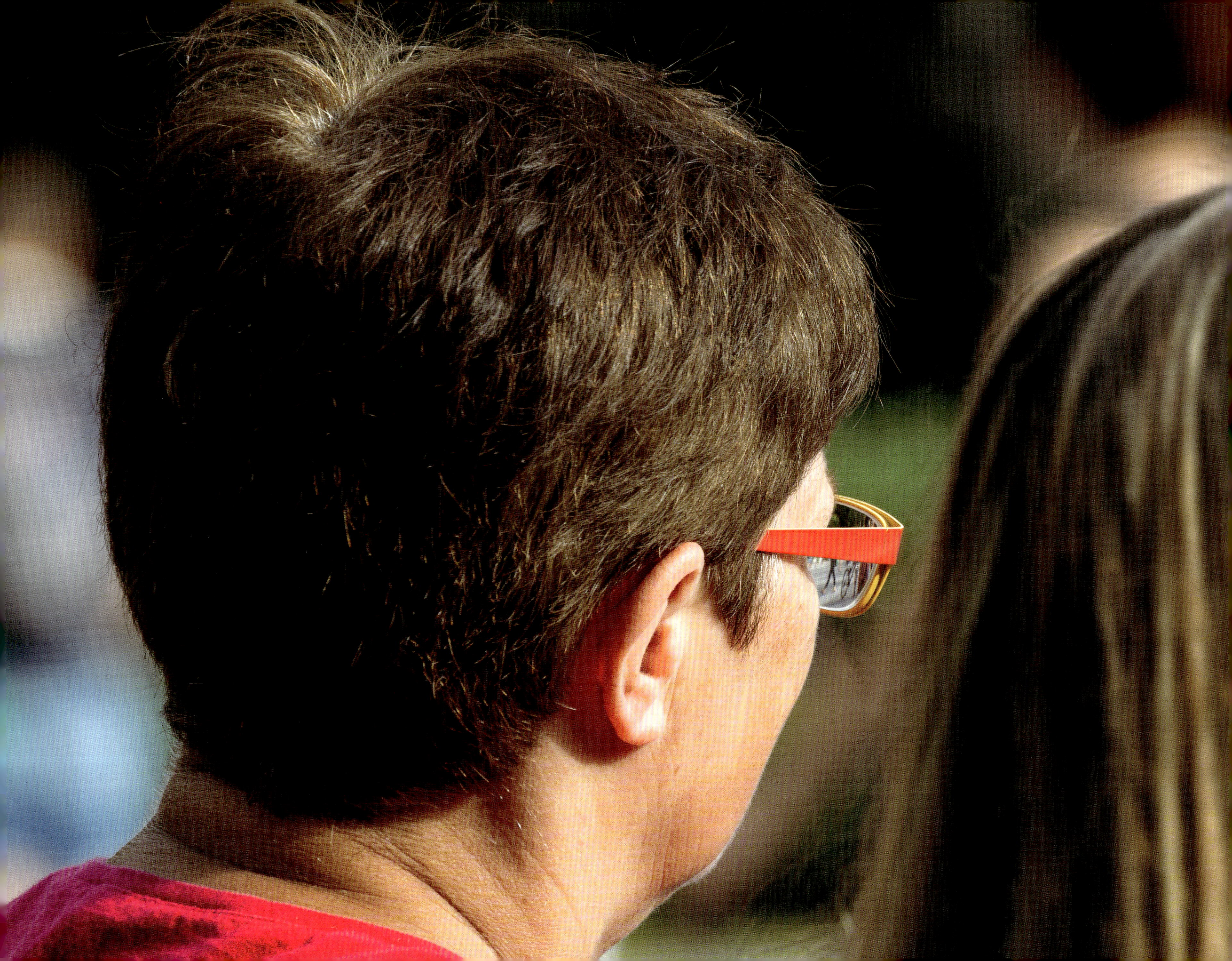

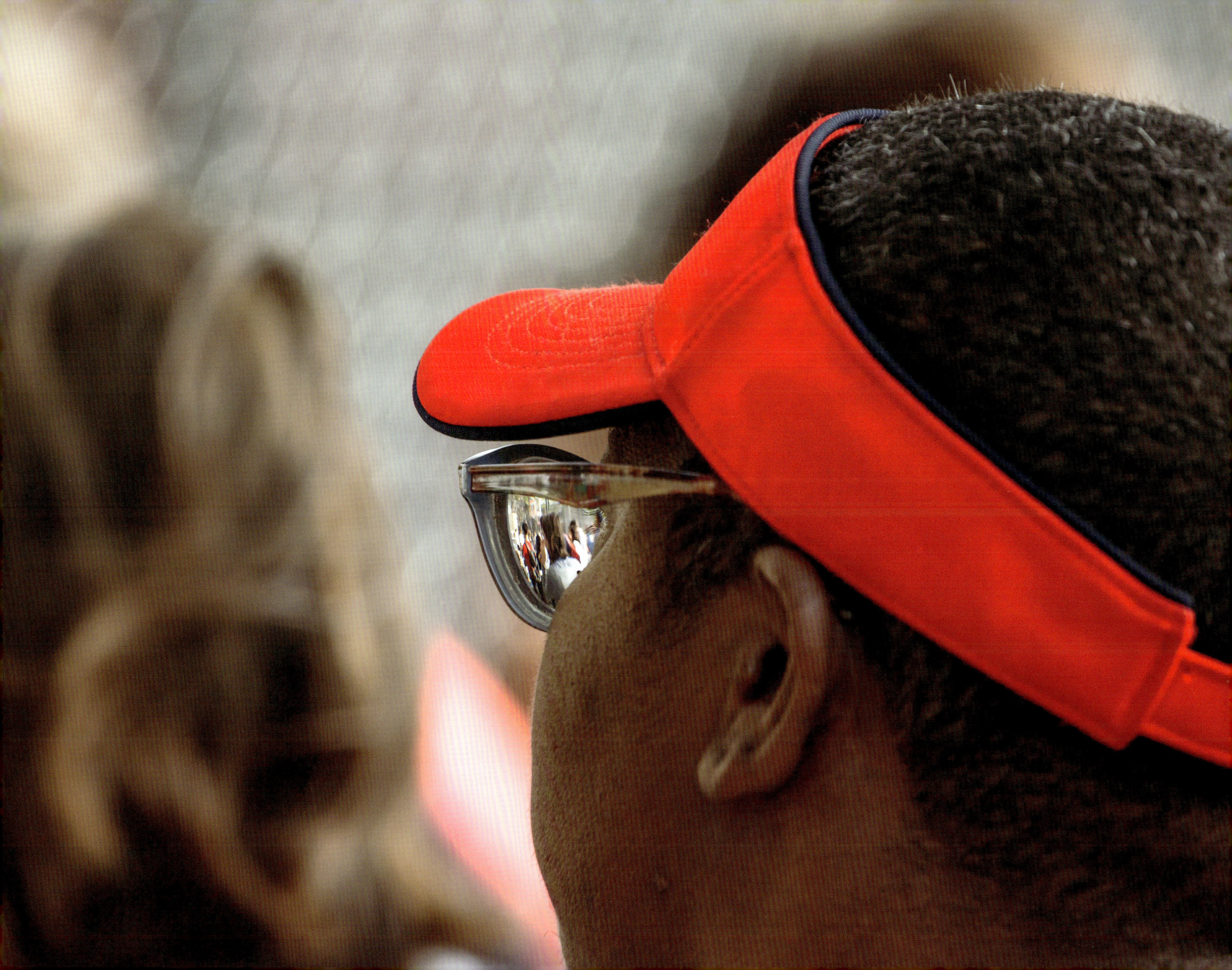

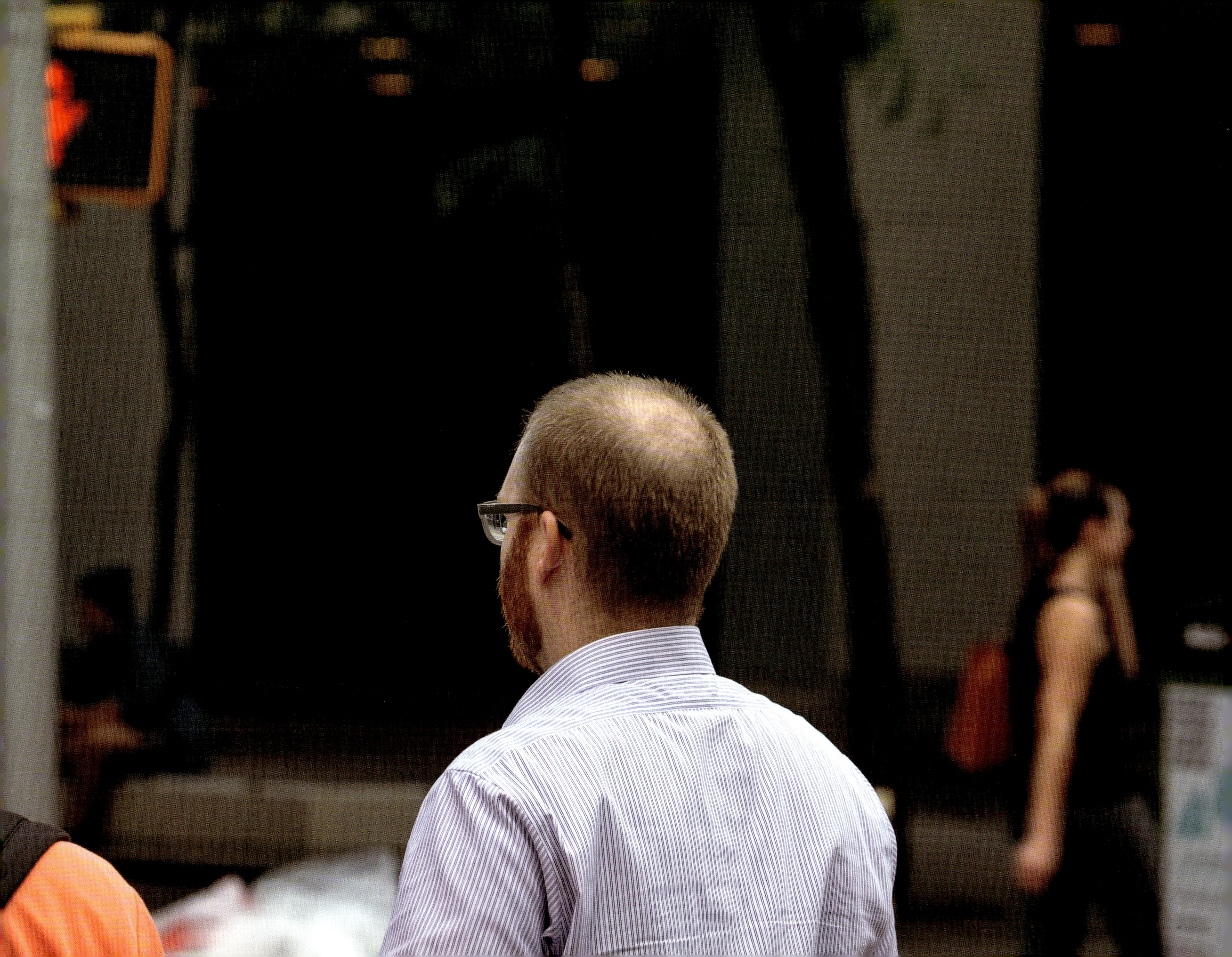

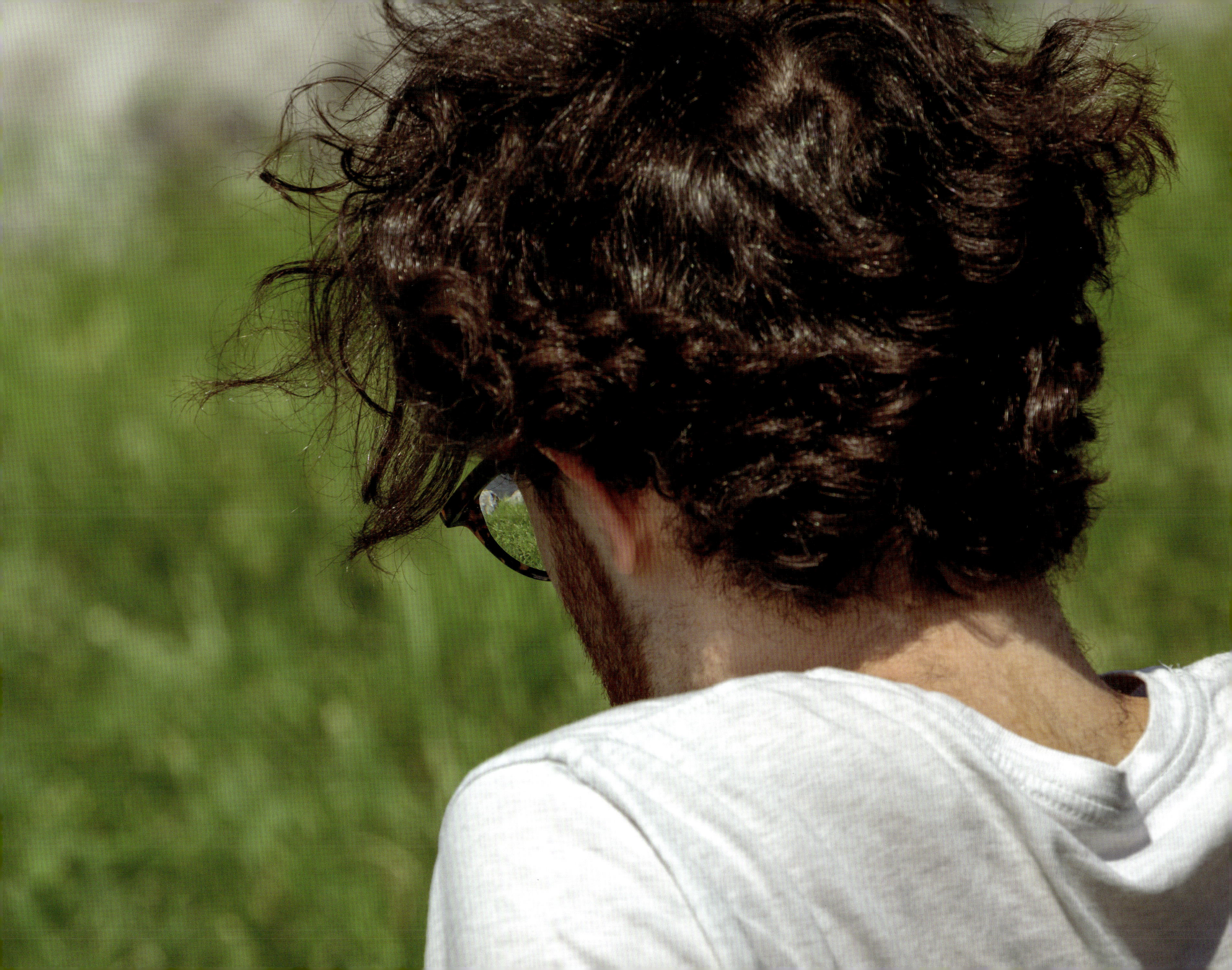

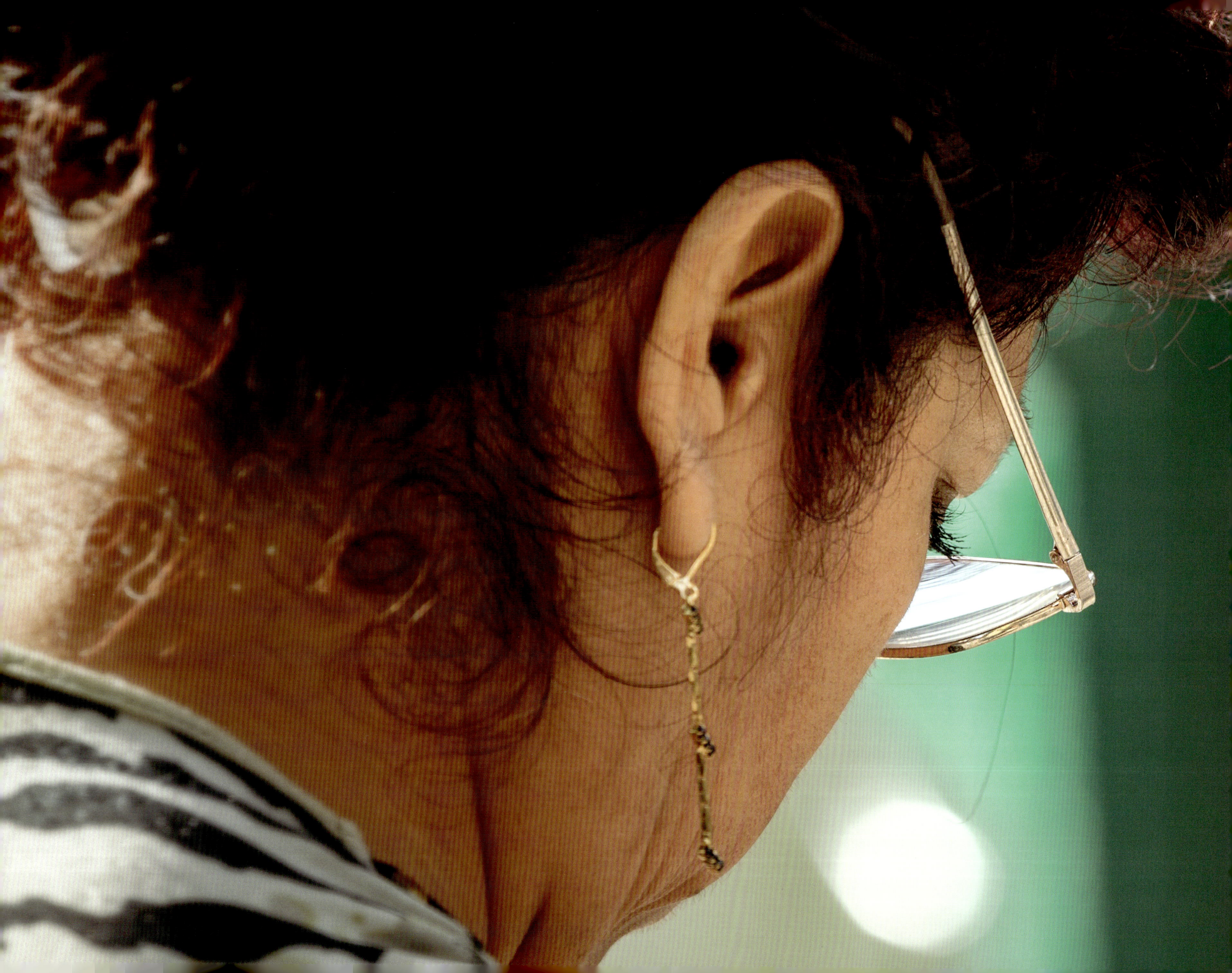

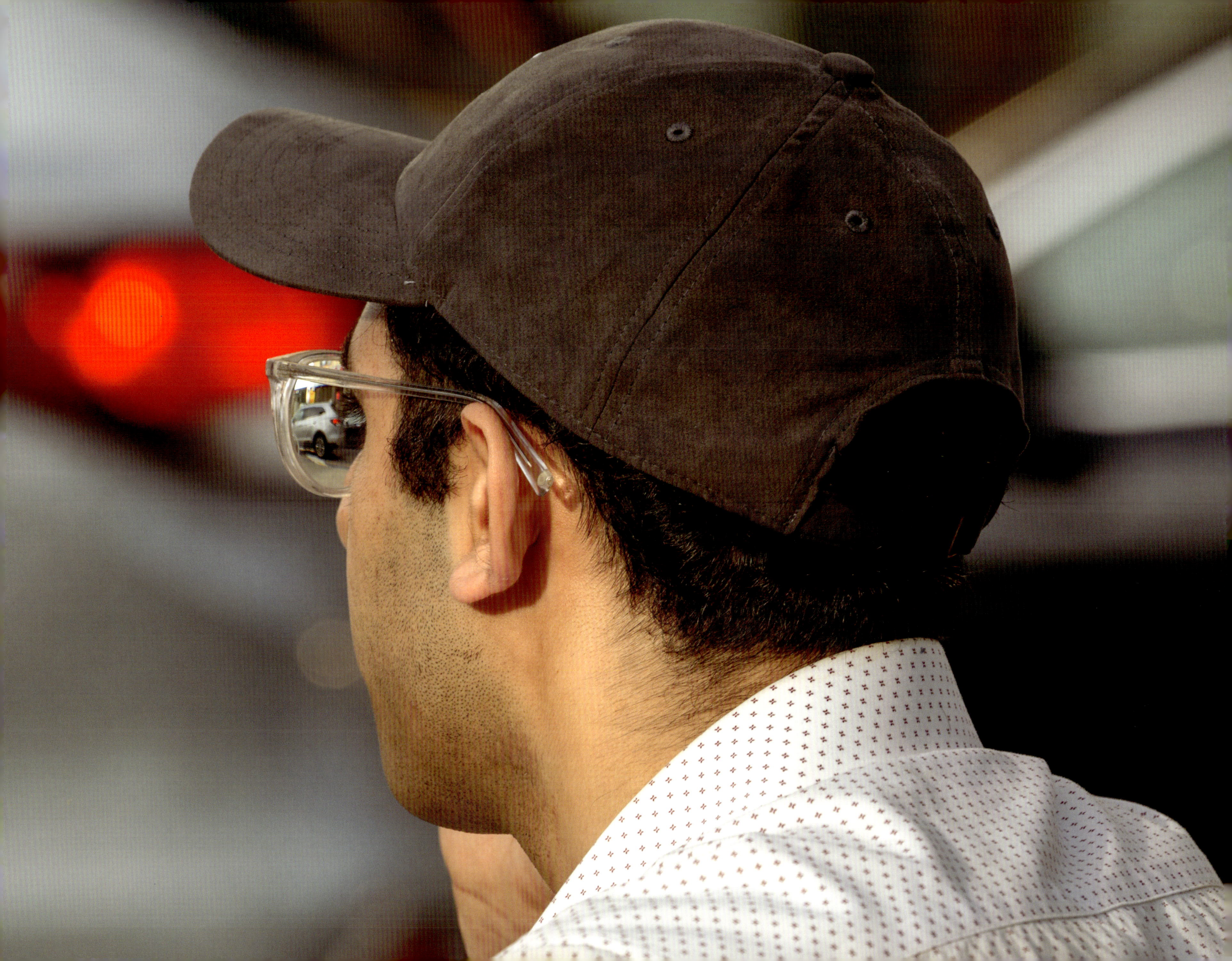

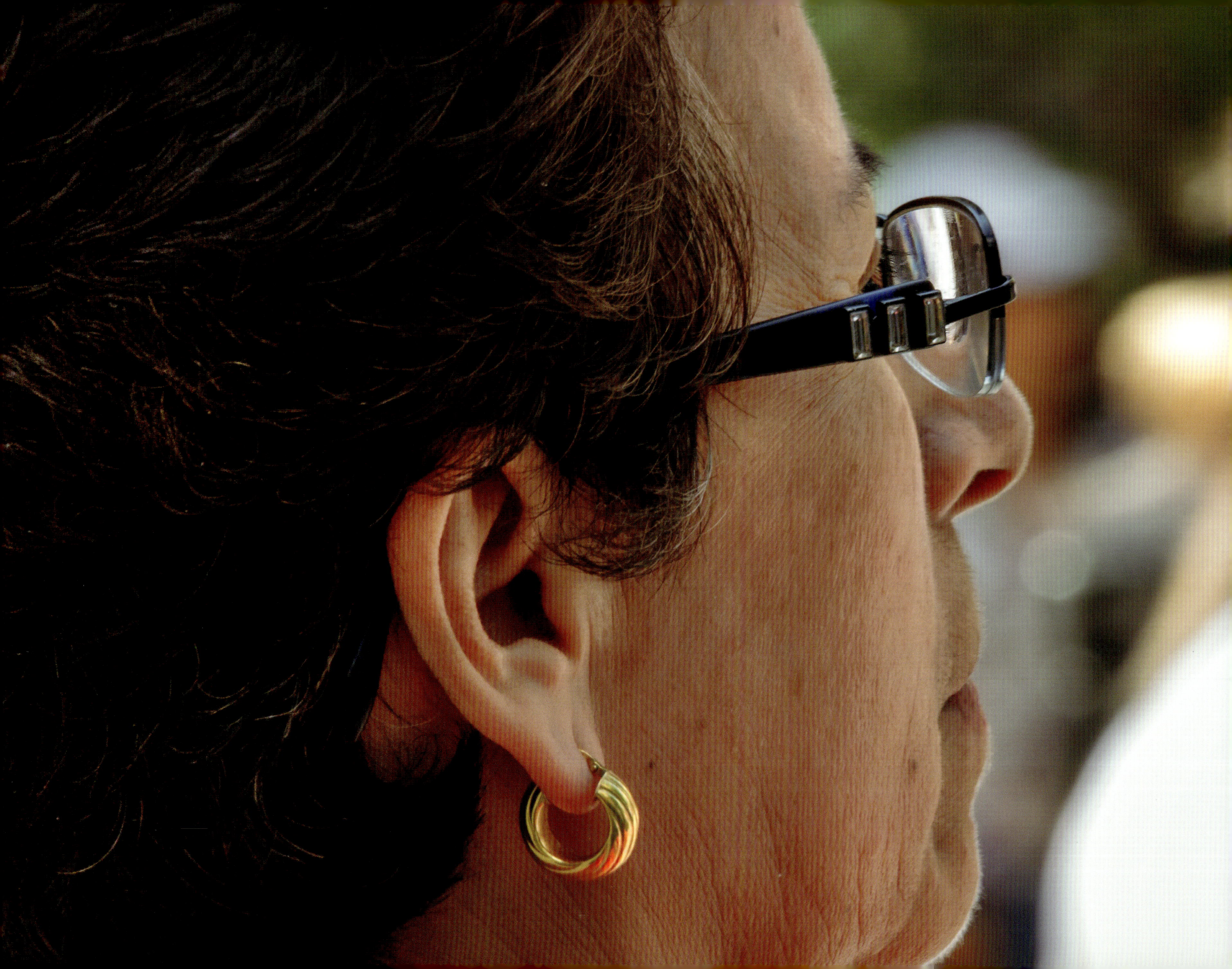

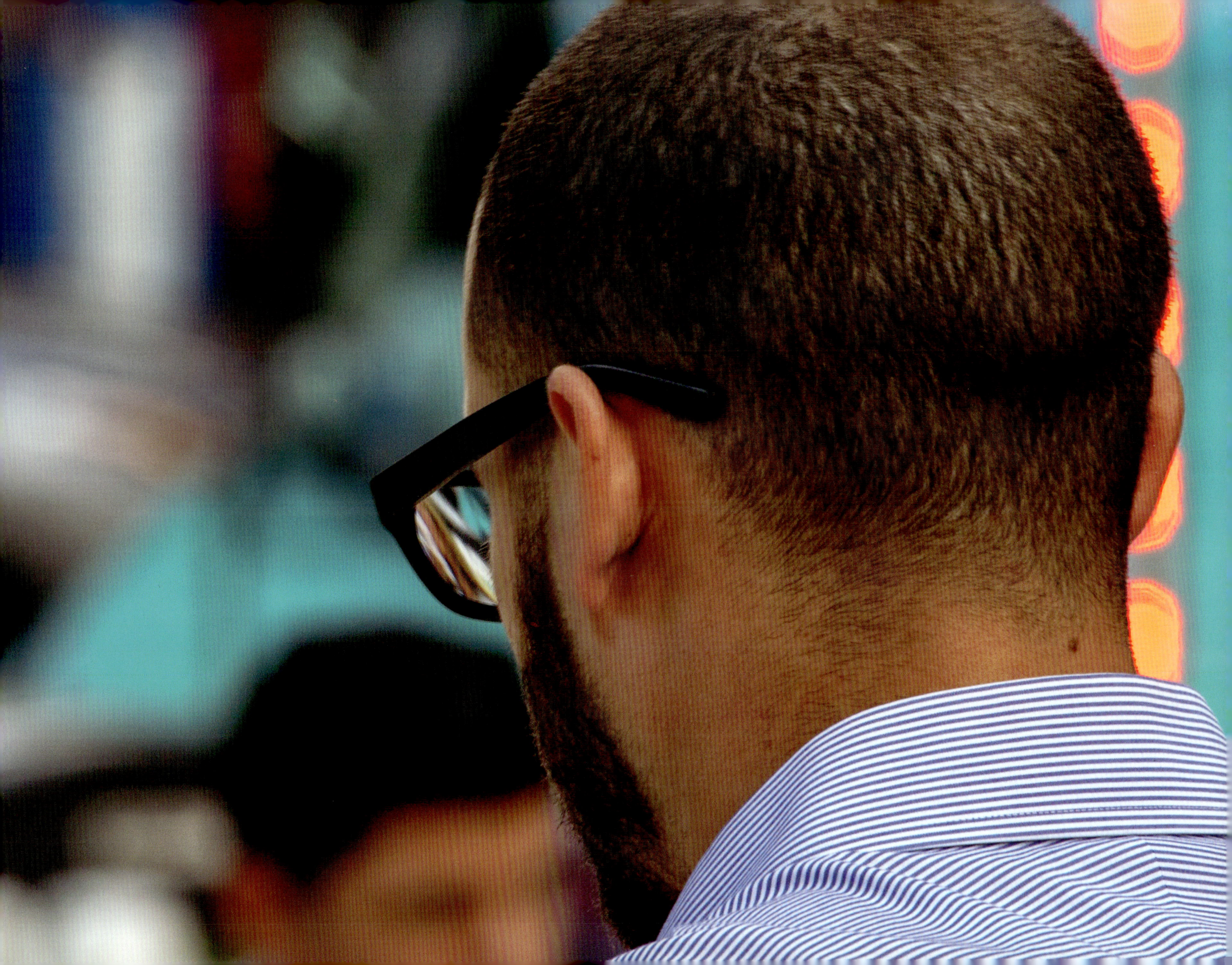

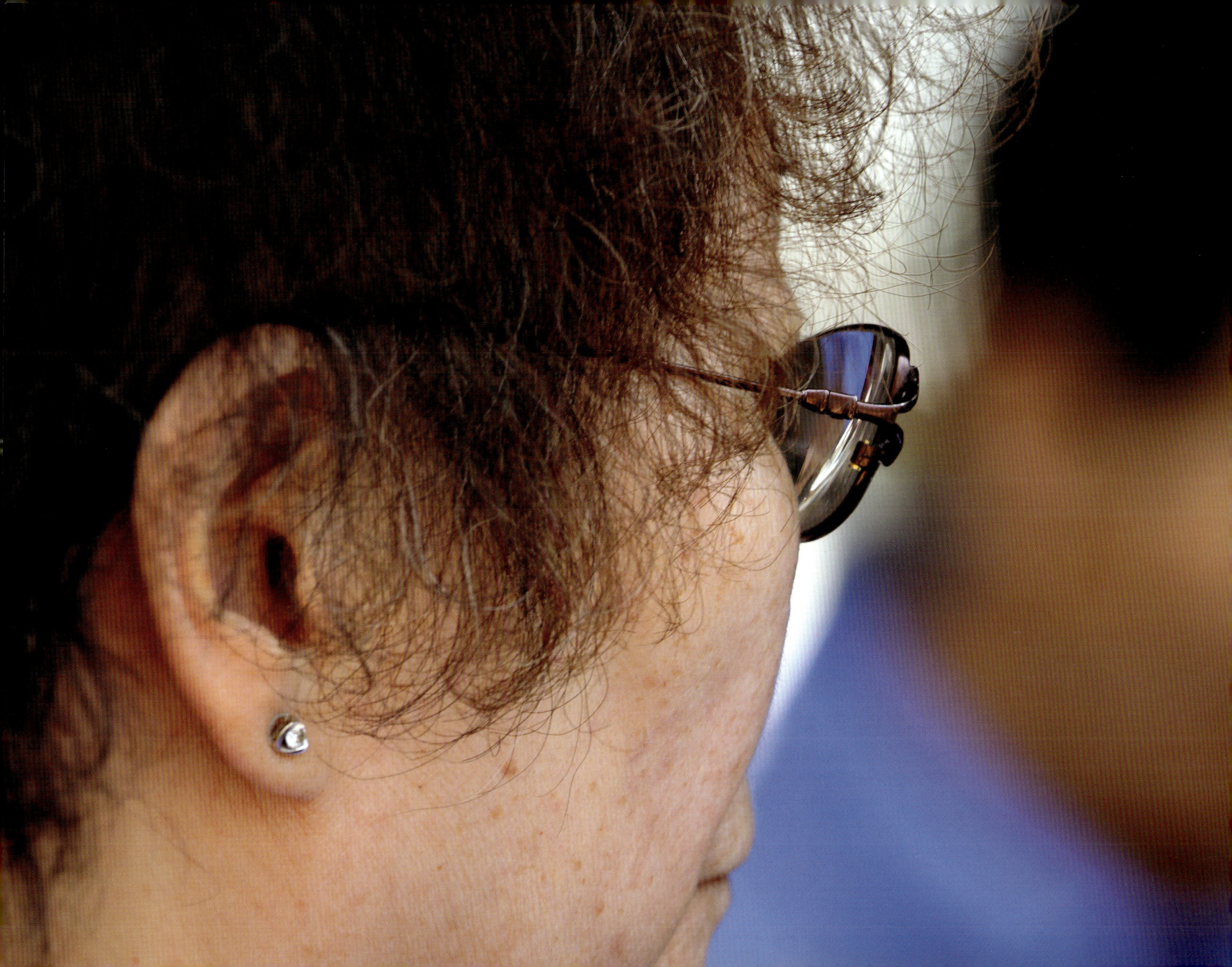

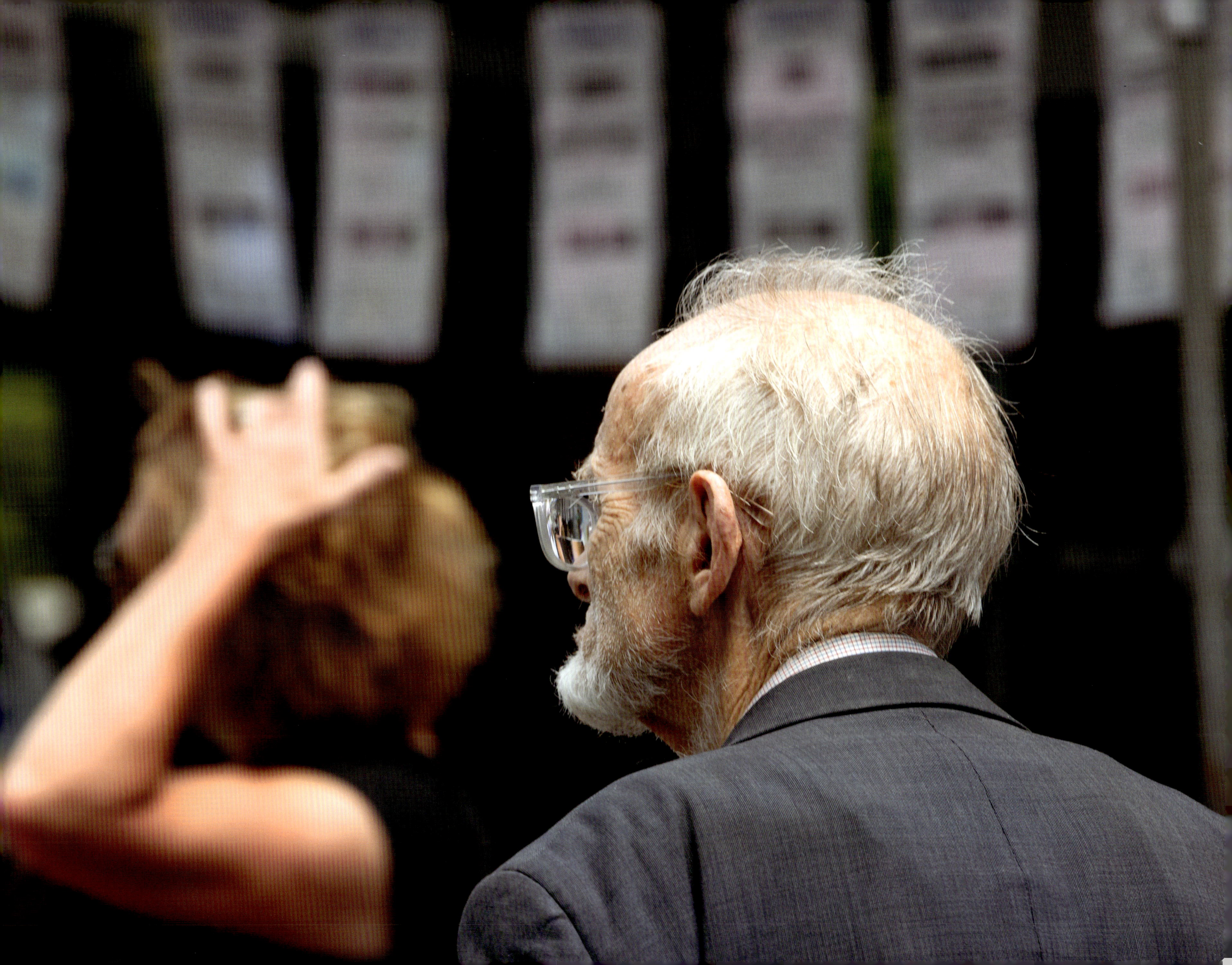

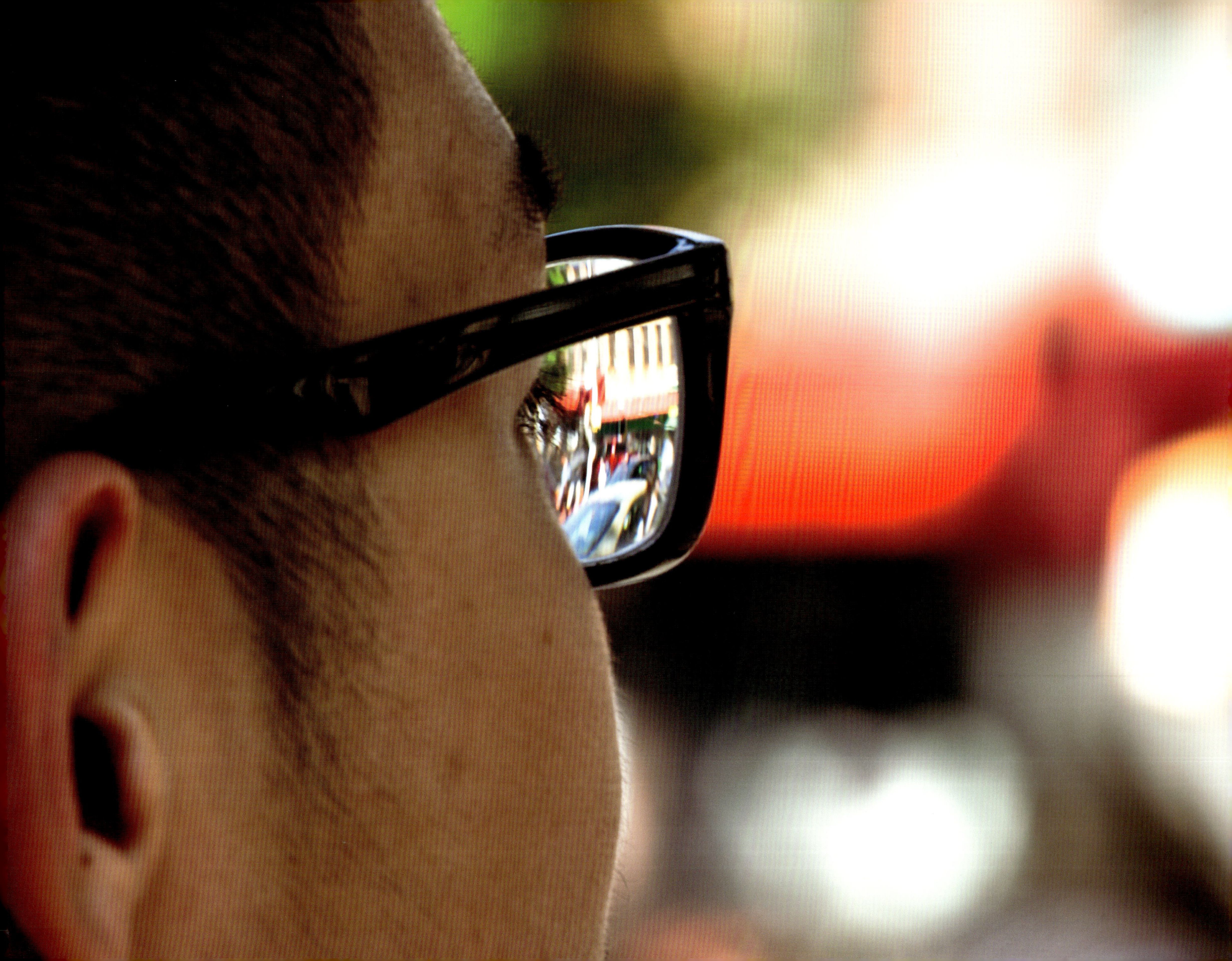

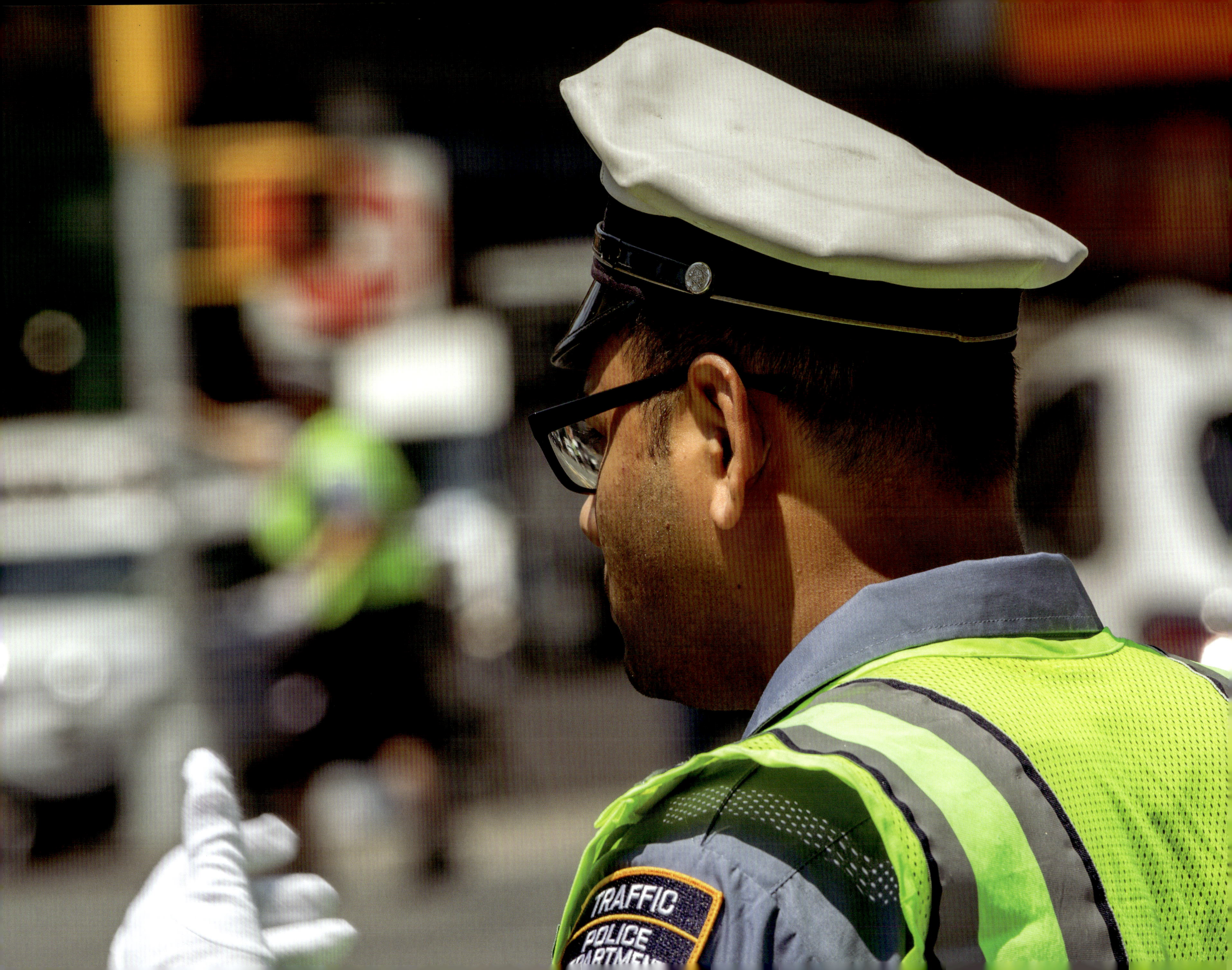

TRAFFIC
POLICE
PARTMEN

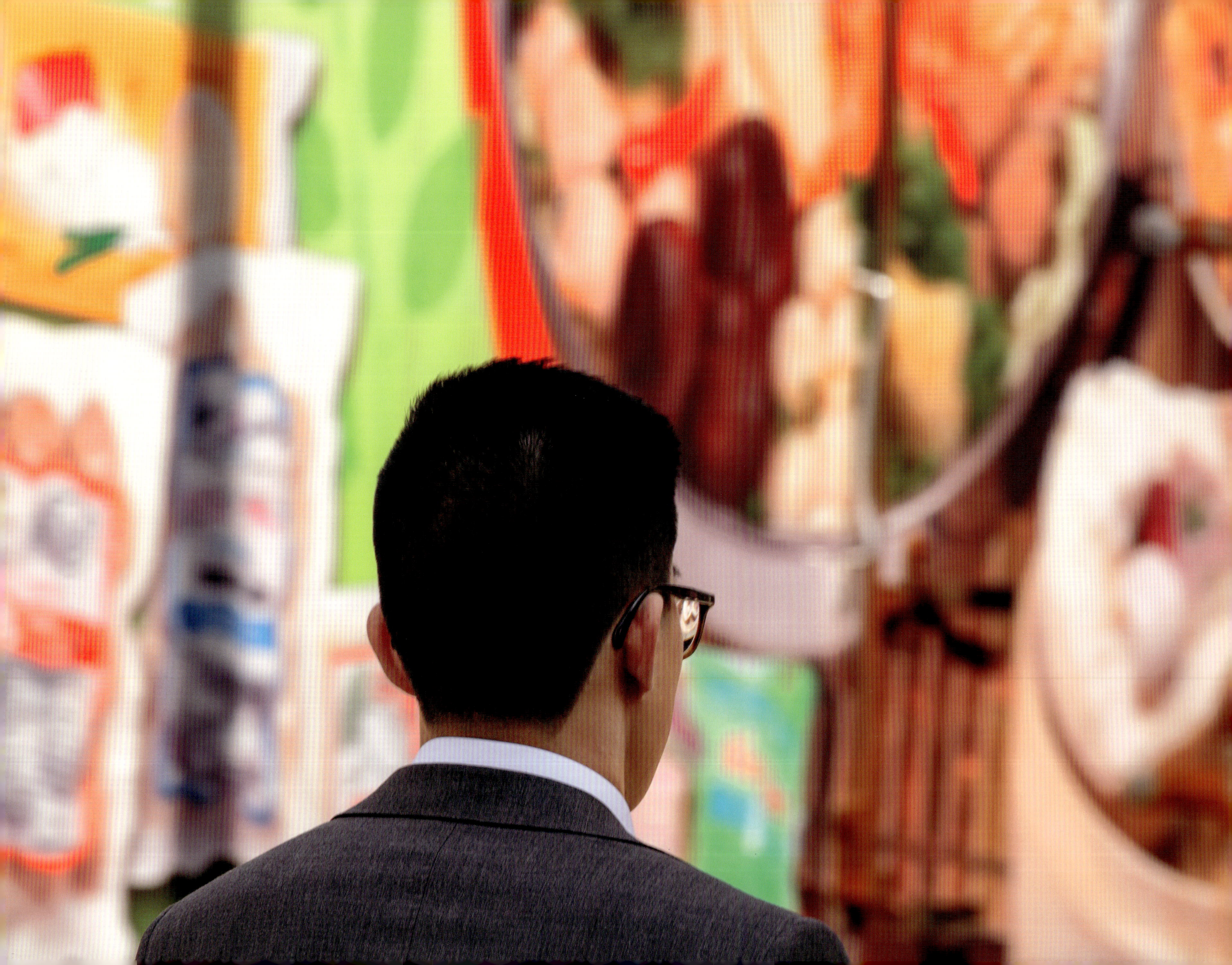

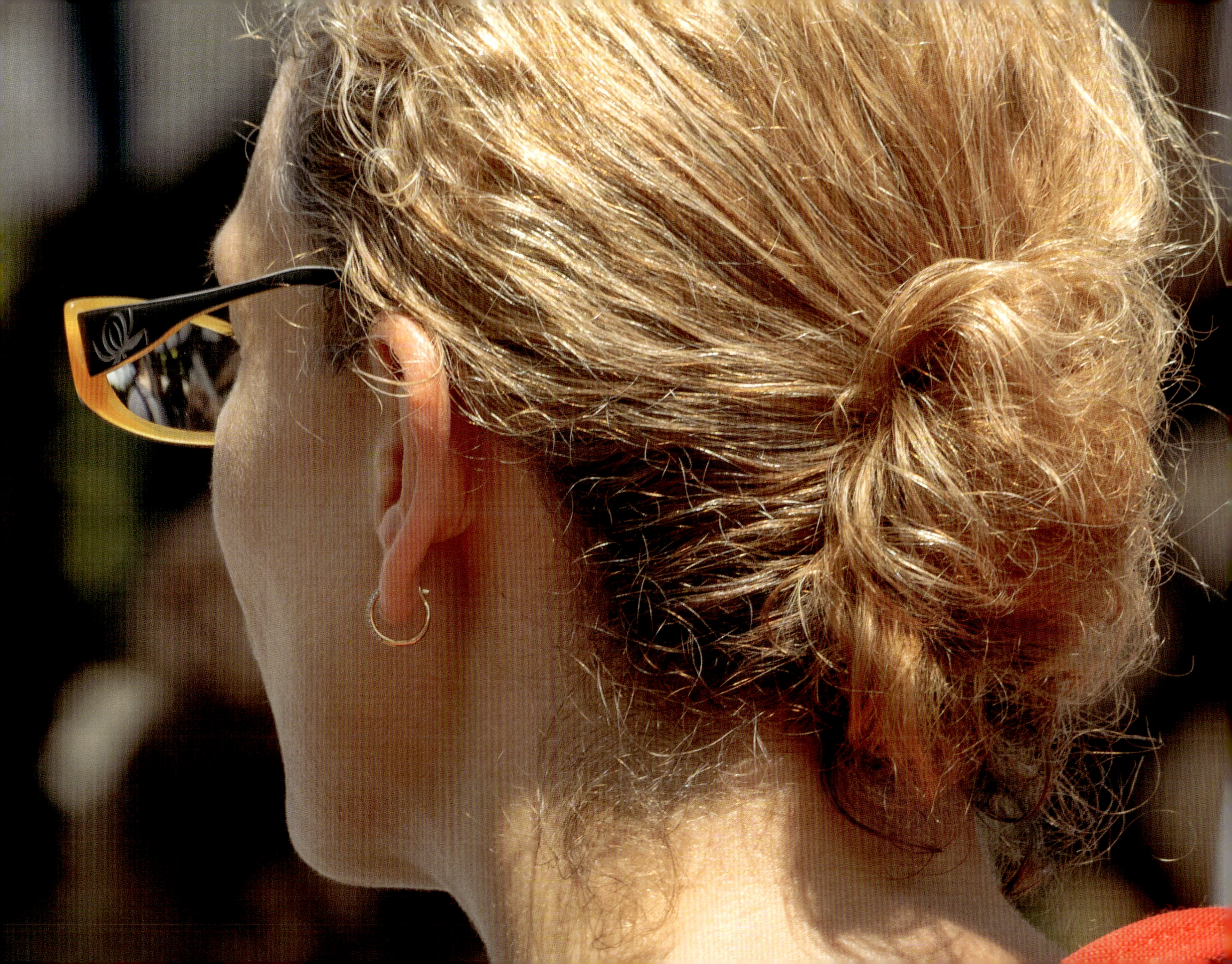

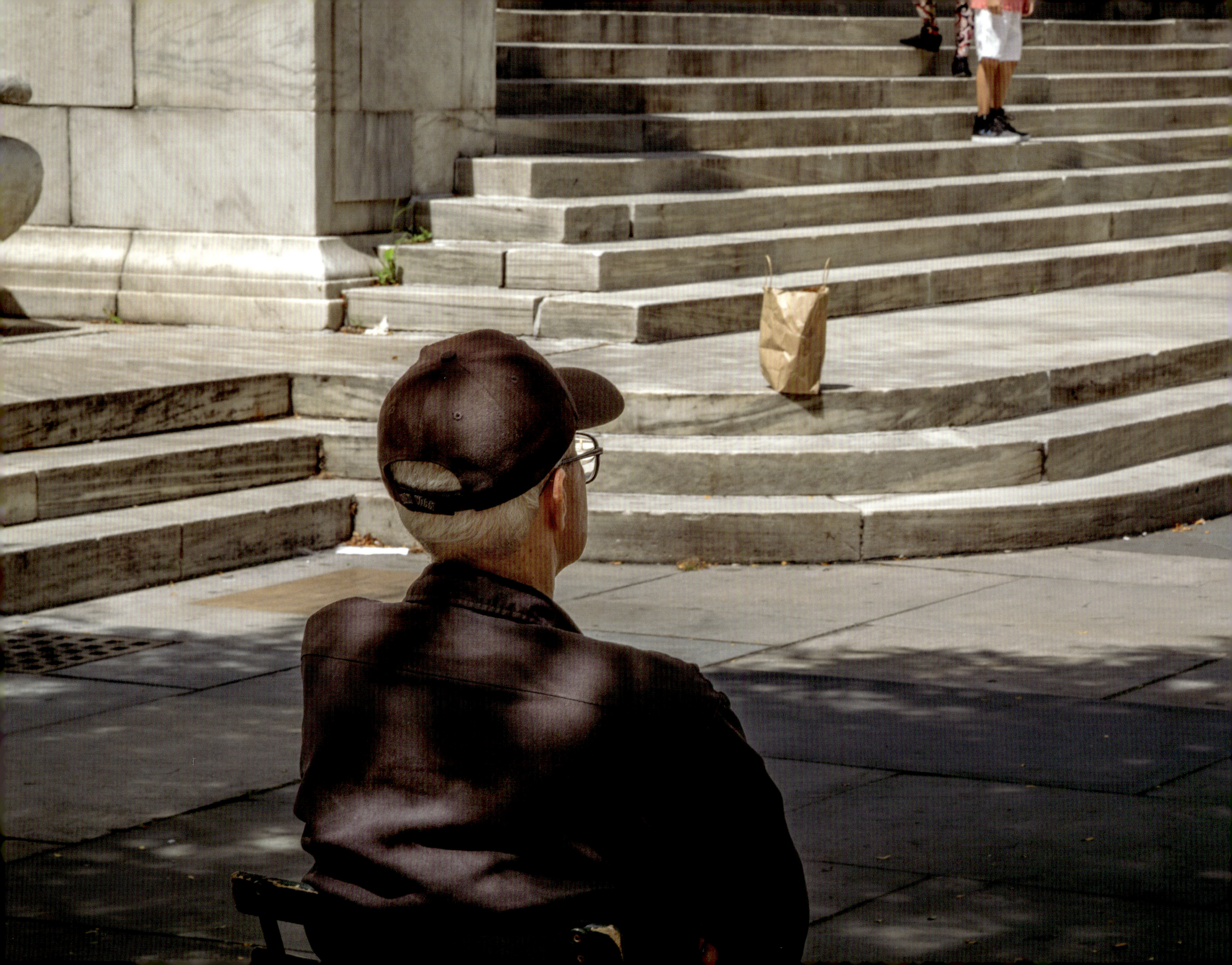

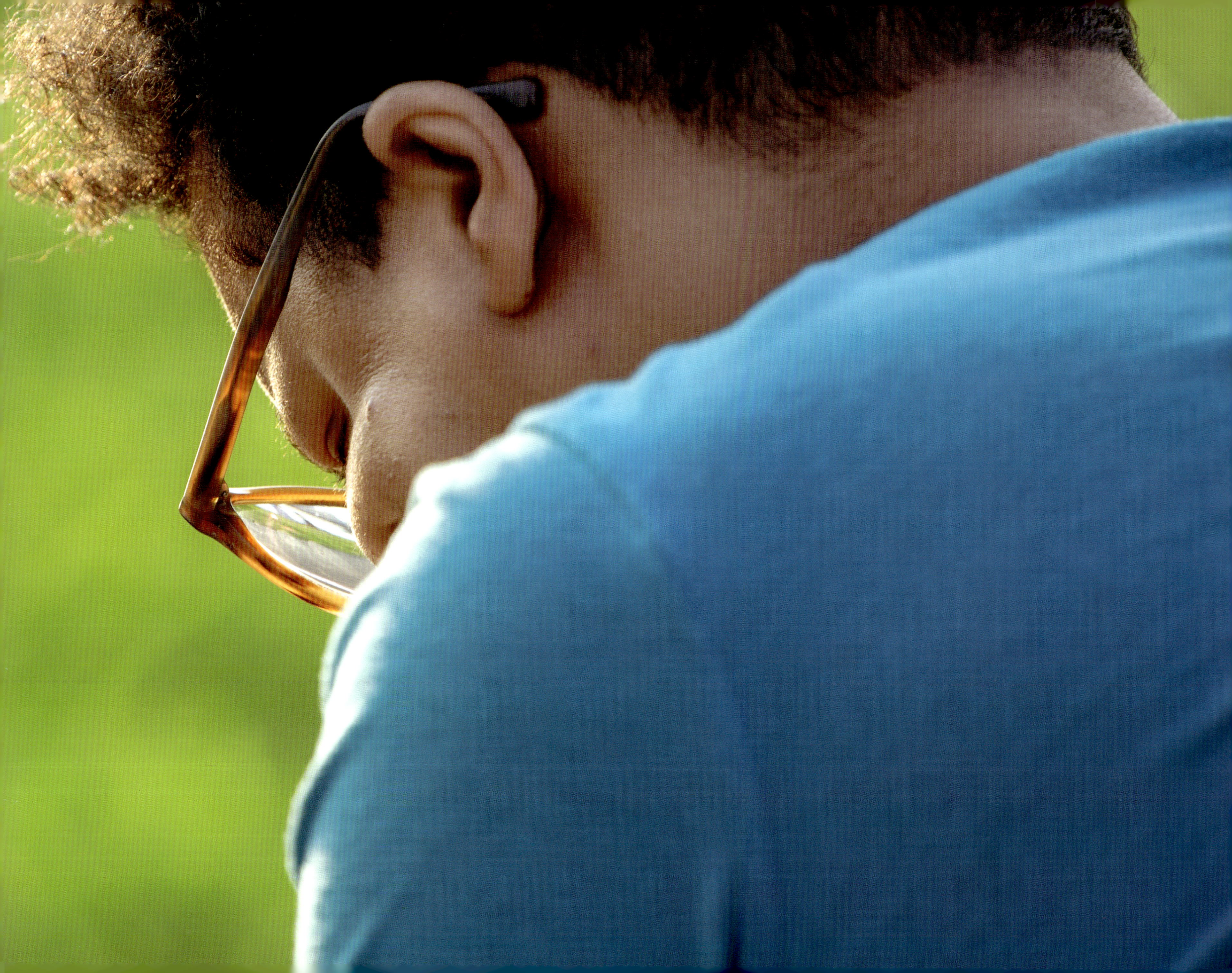

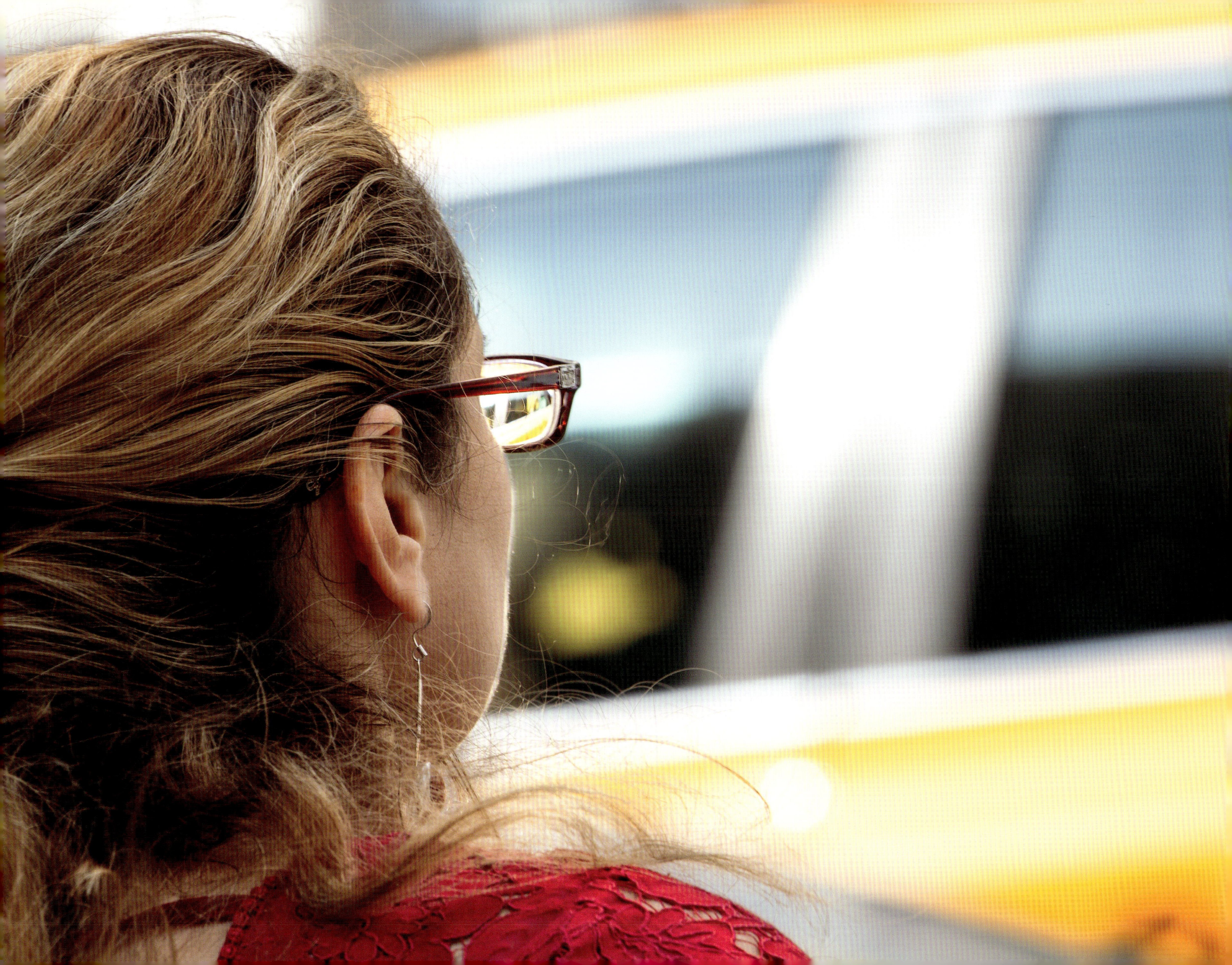

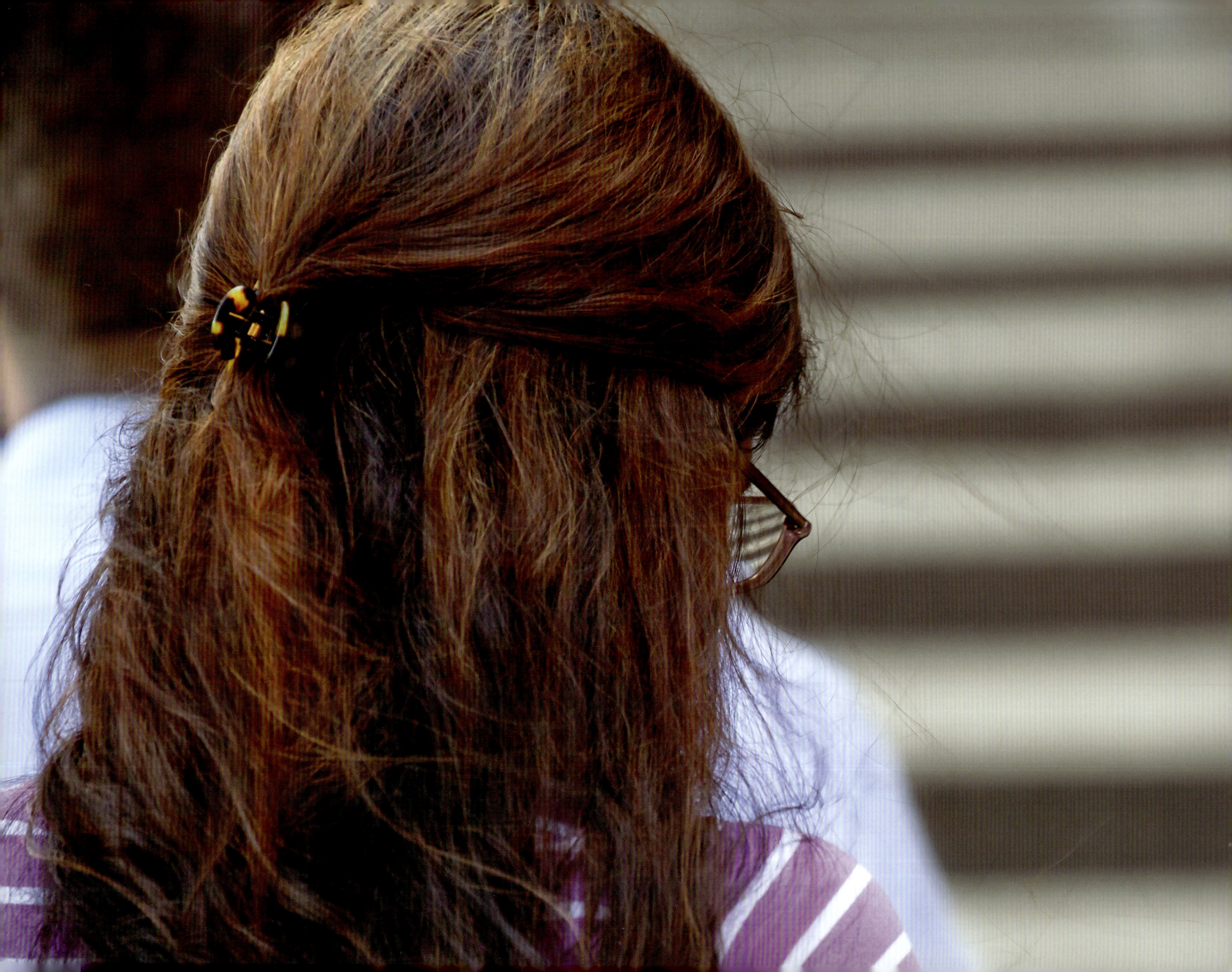

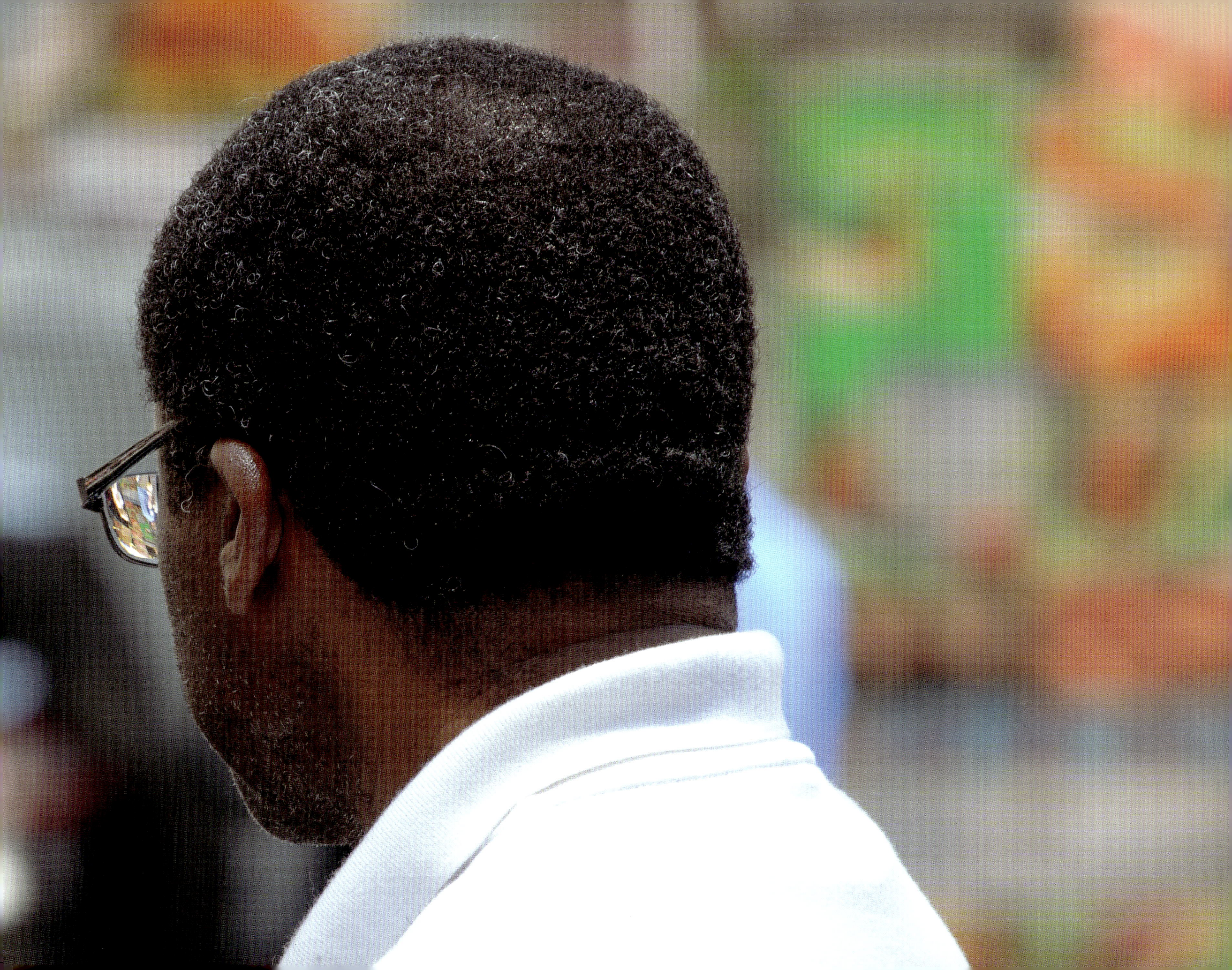

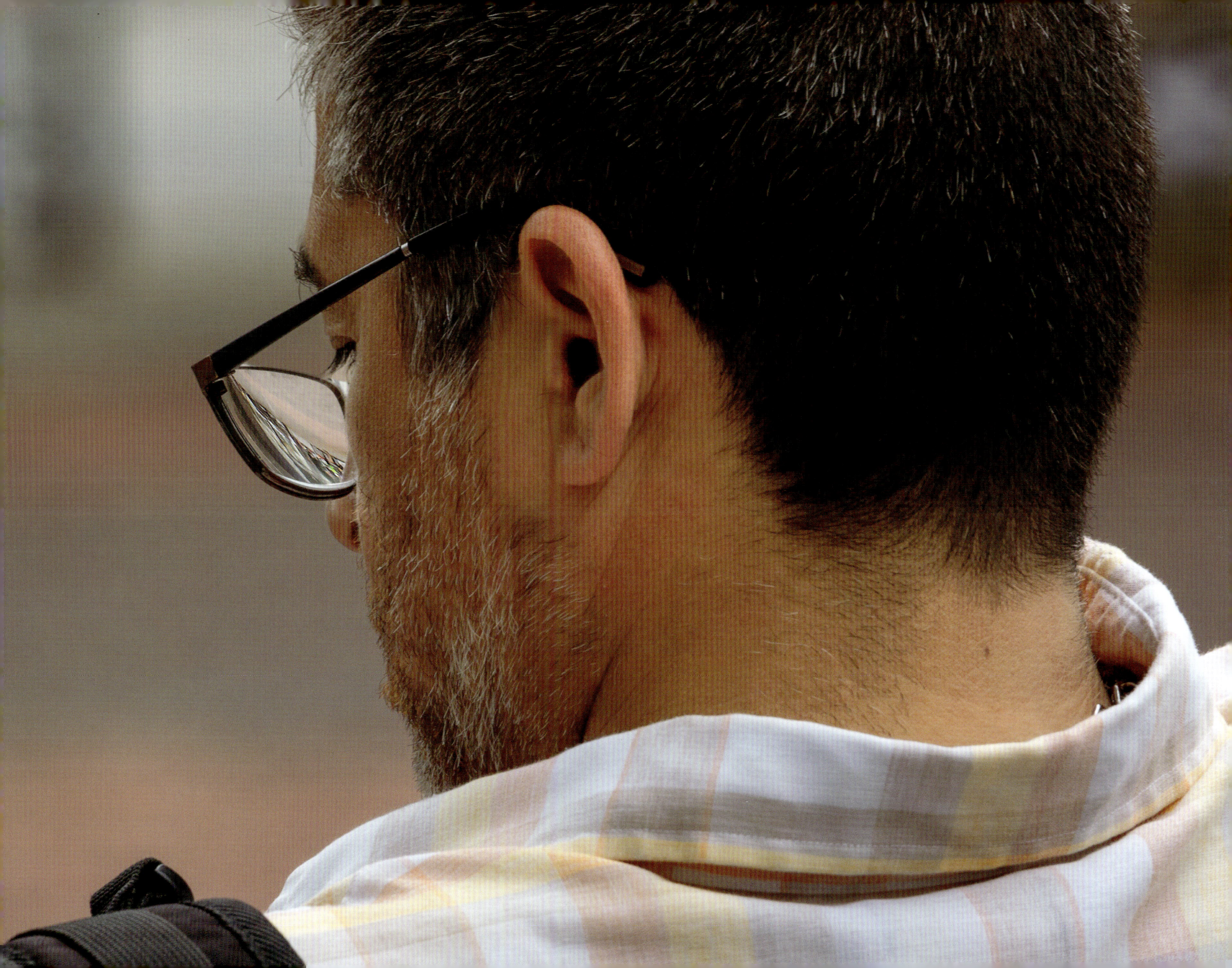

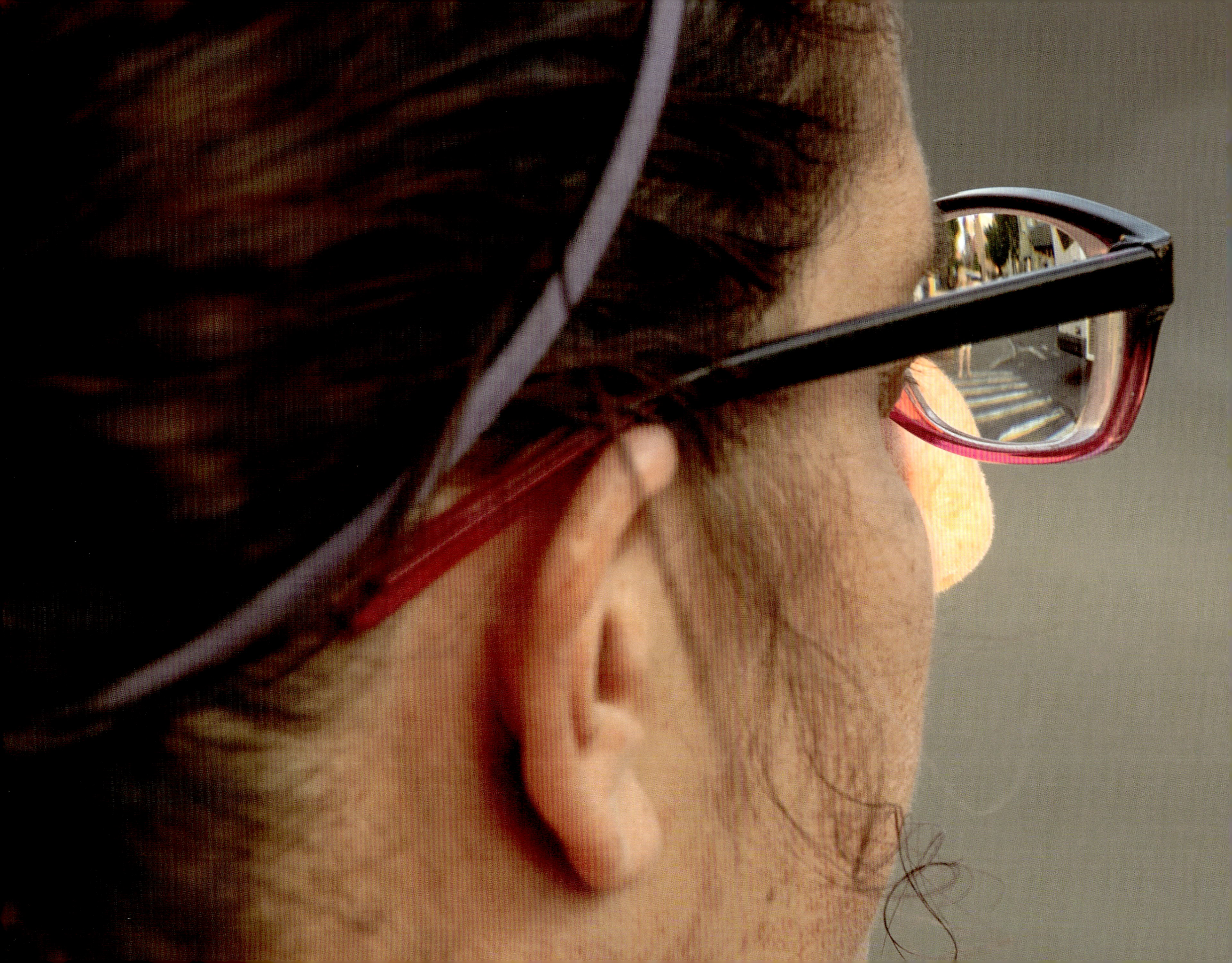

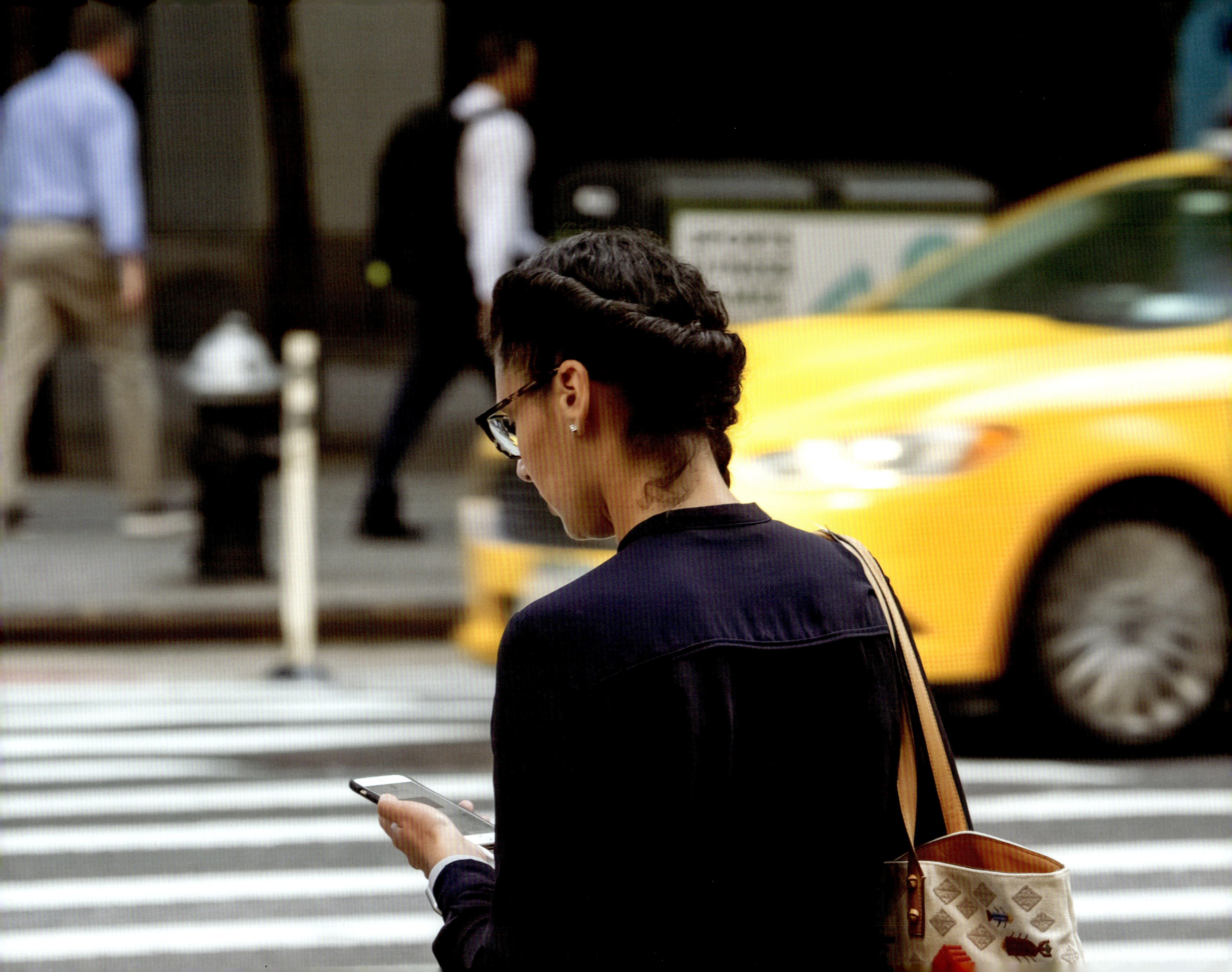

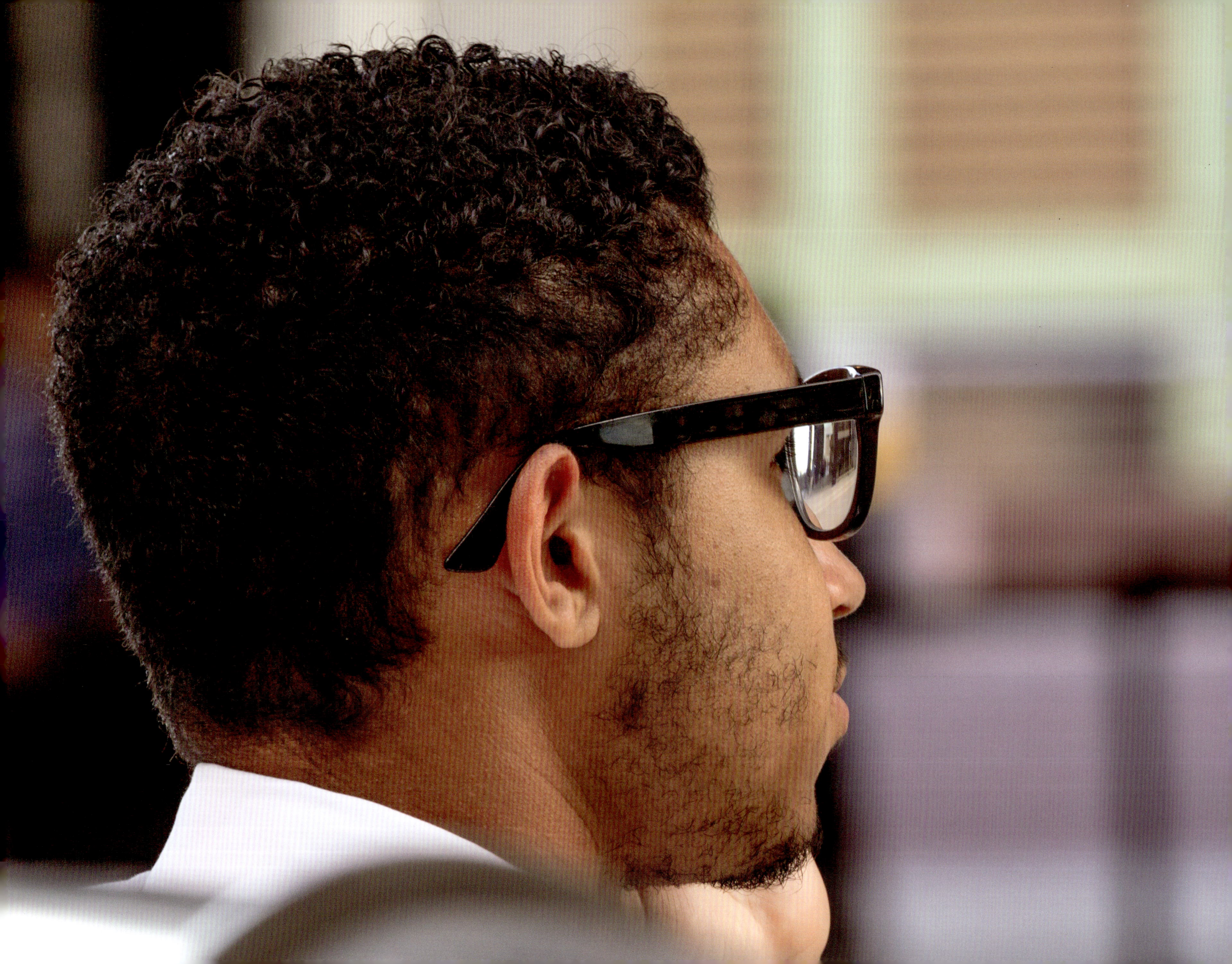

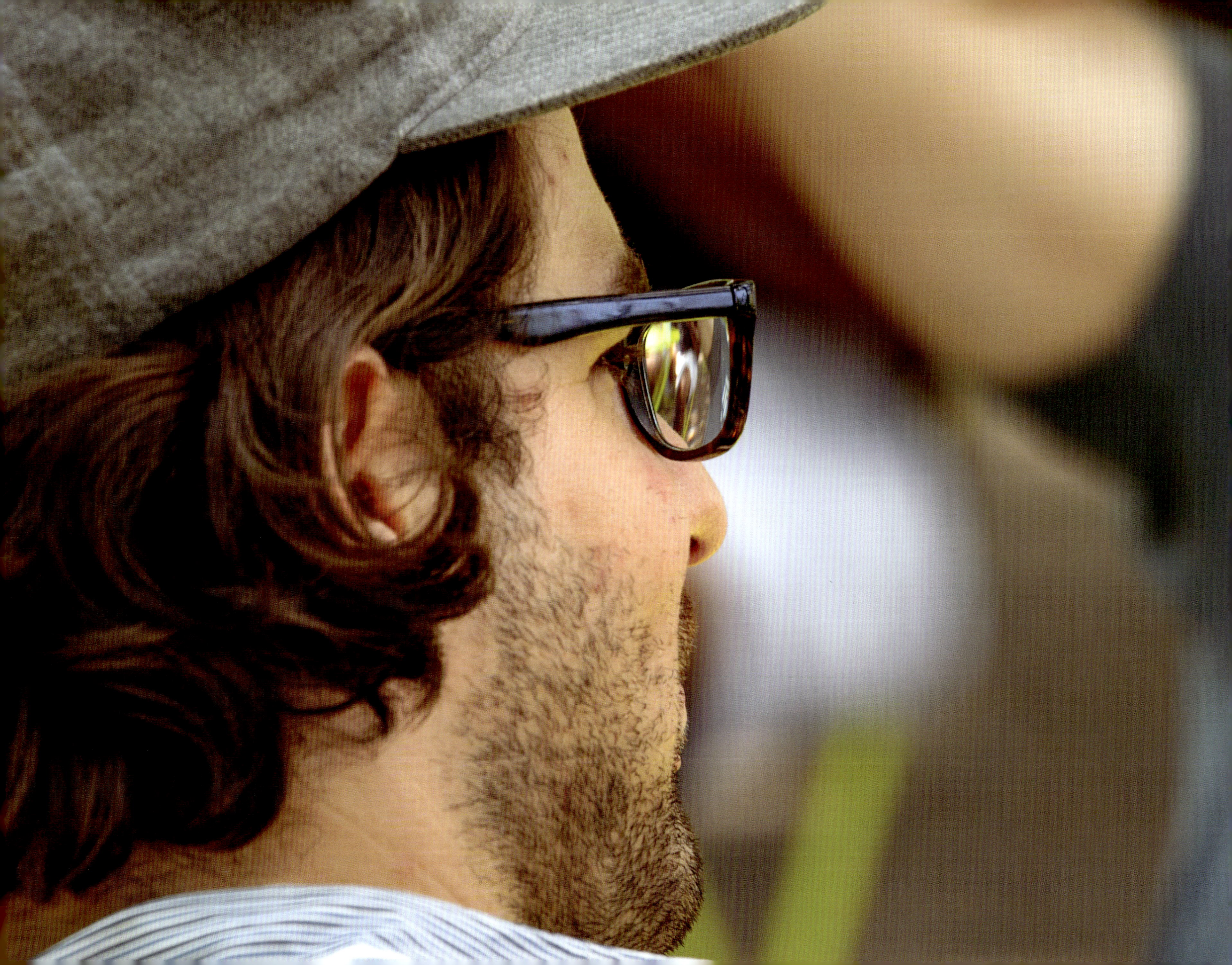

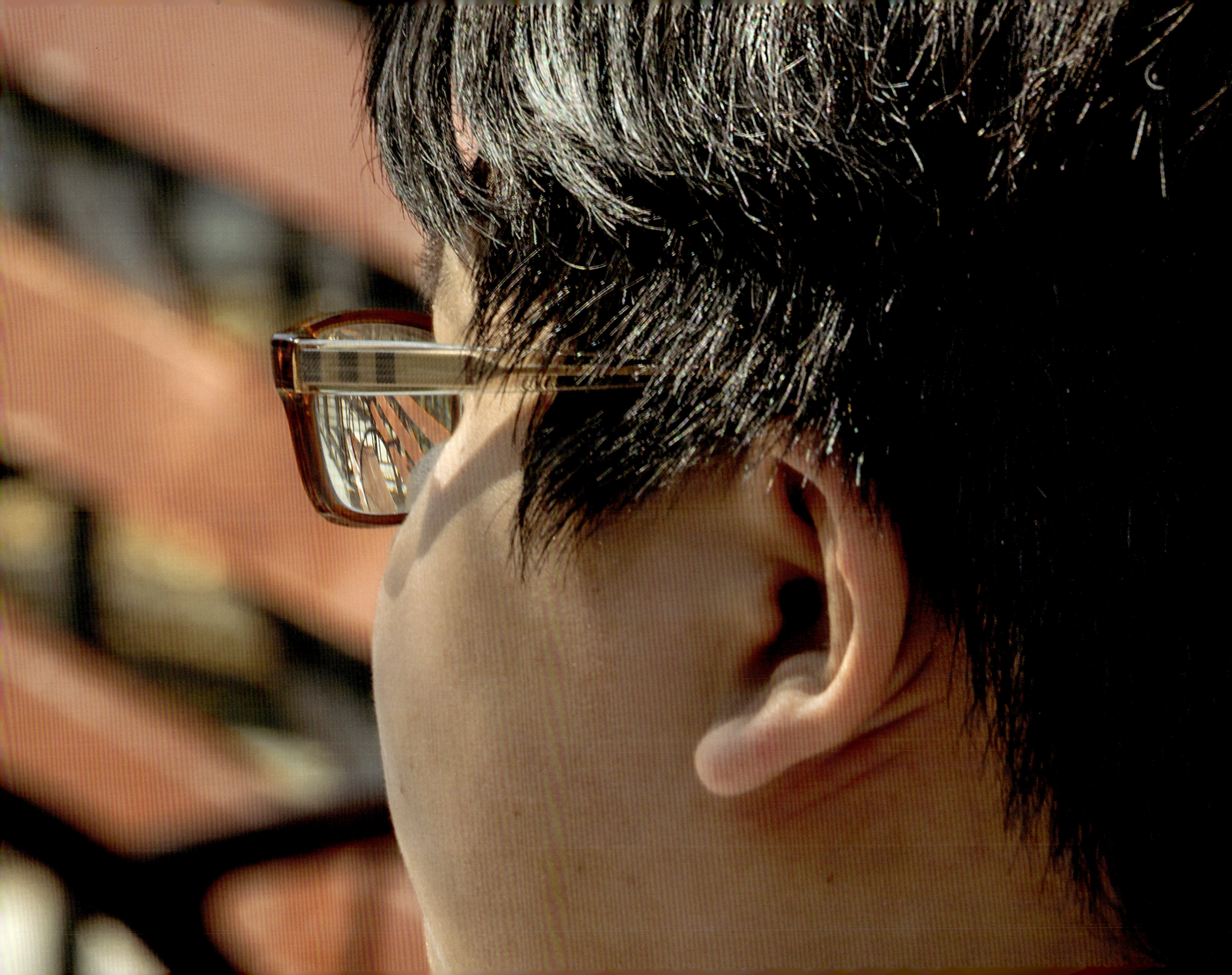

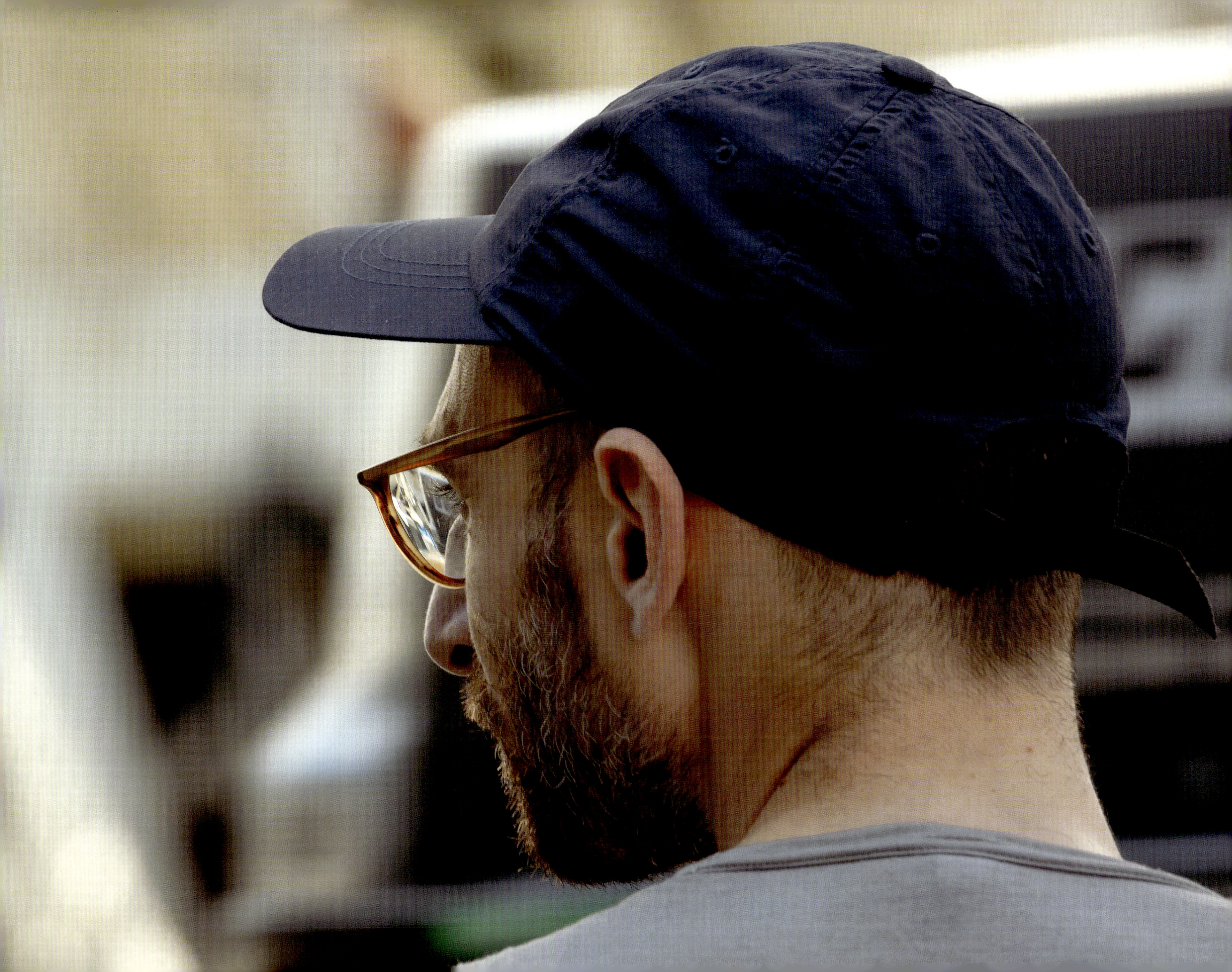

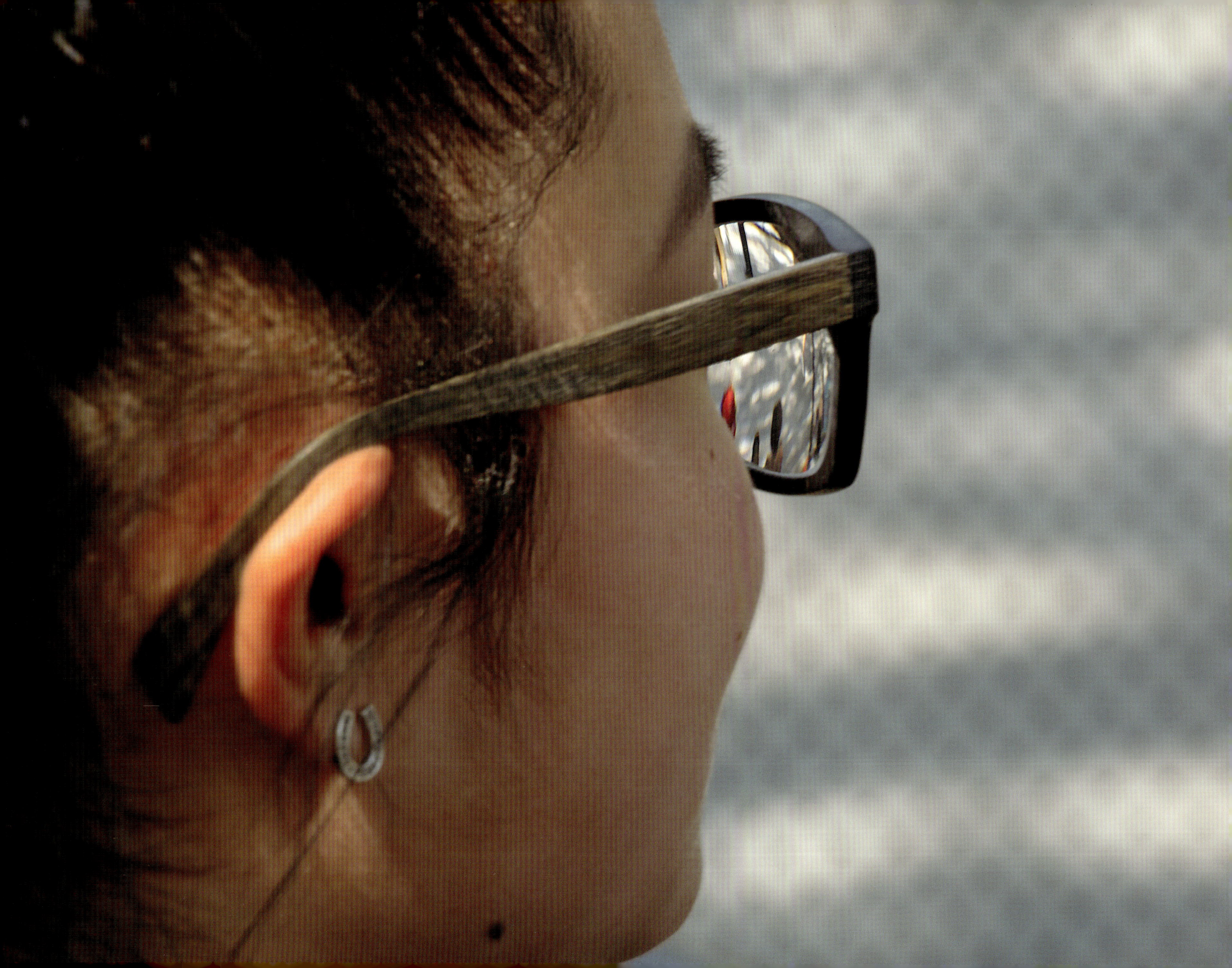

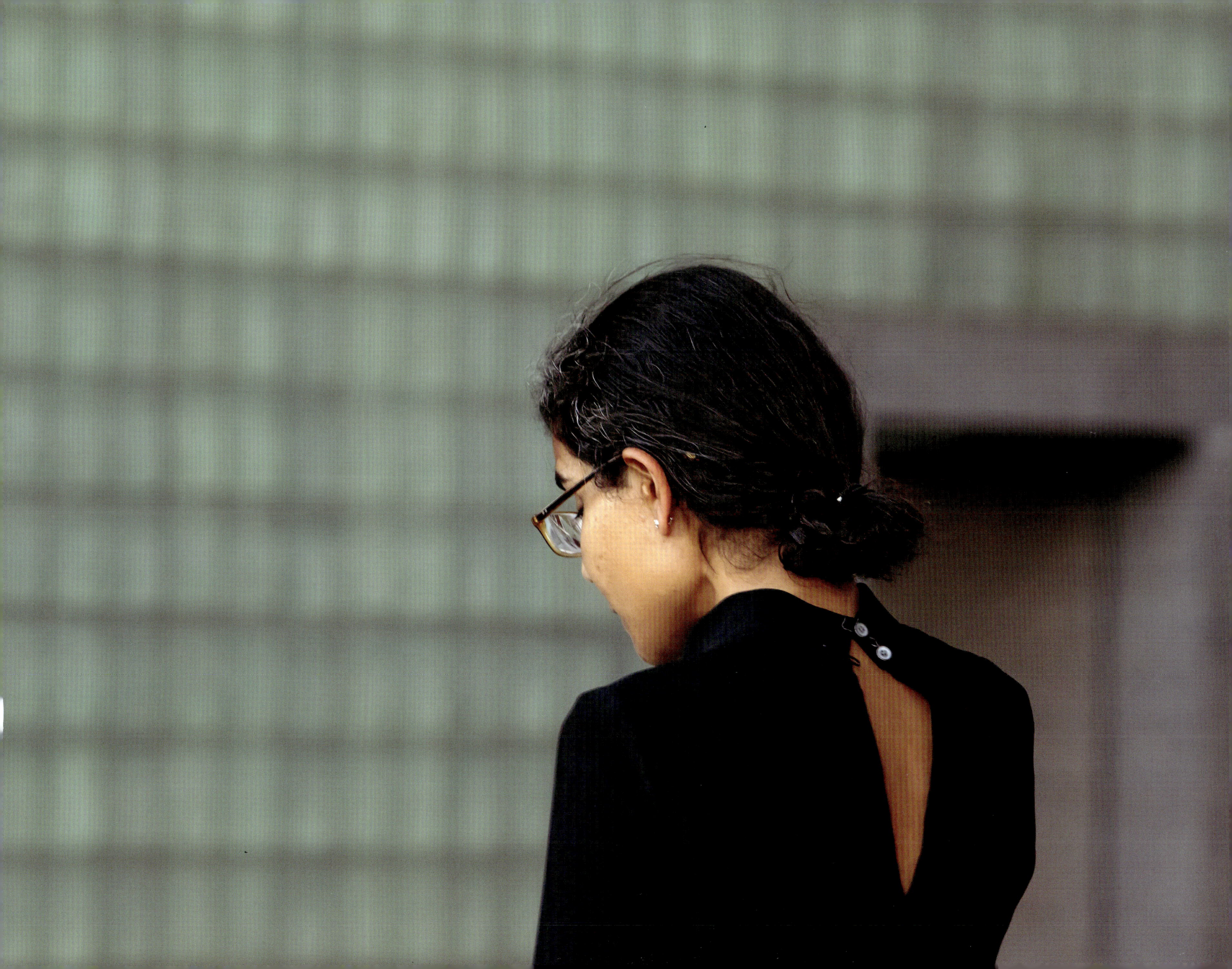

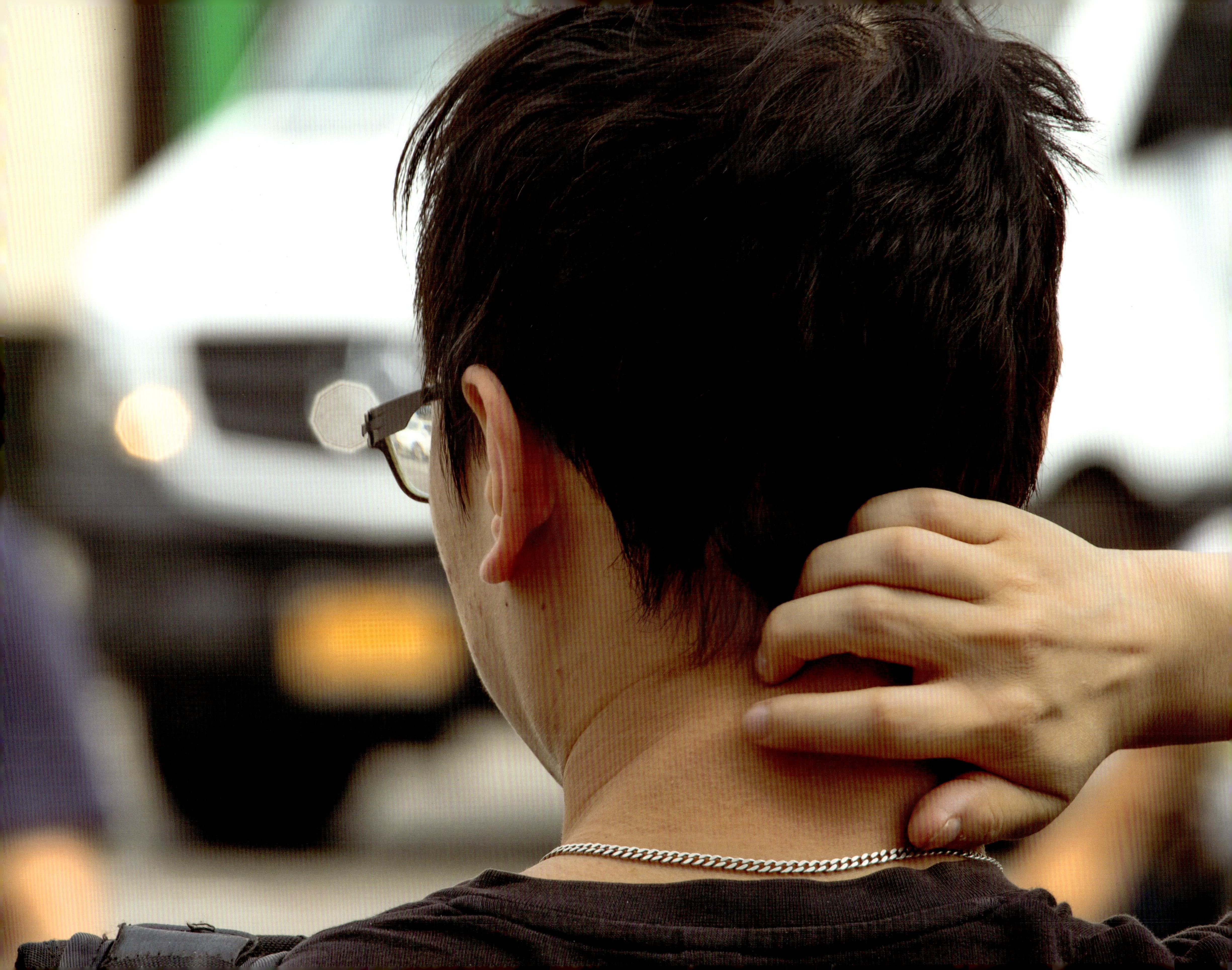

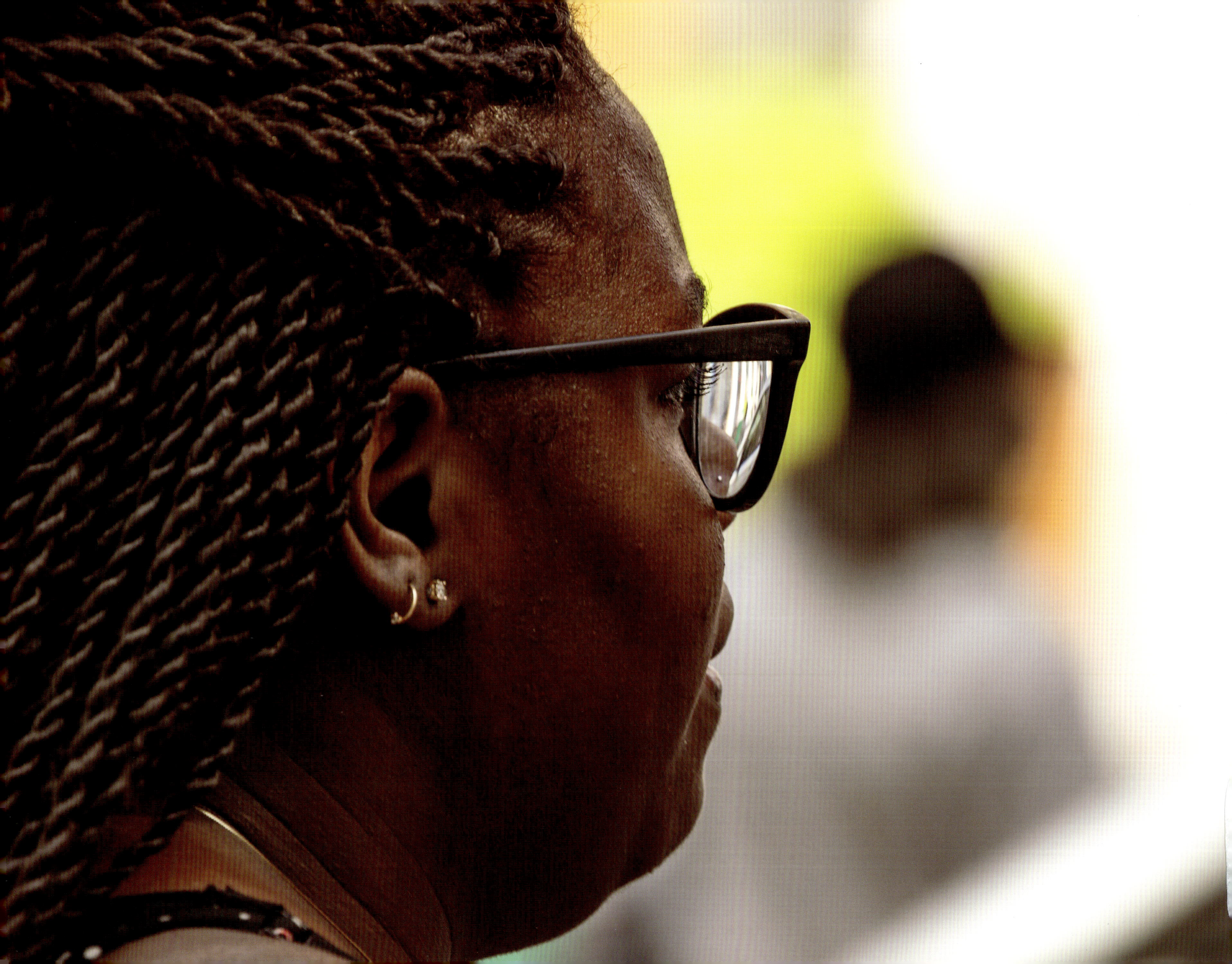

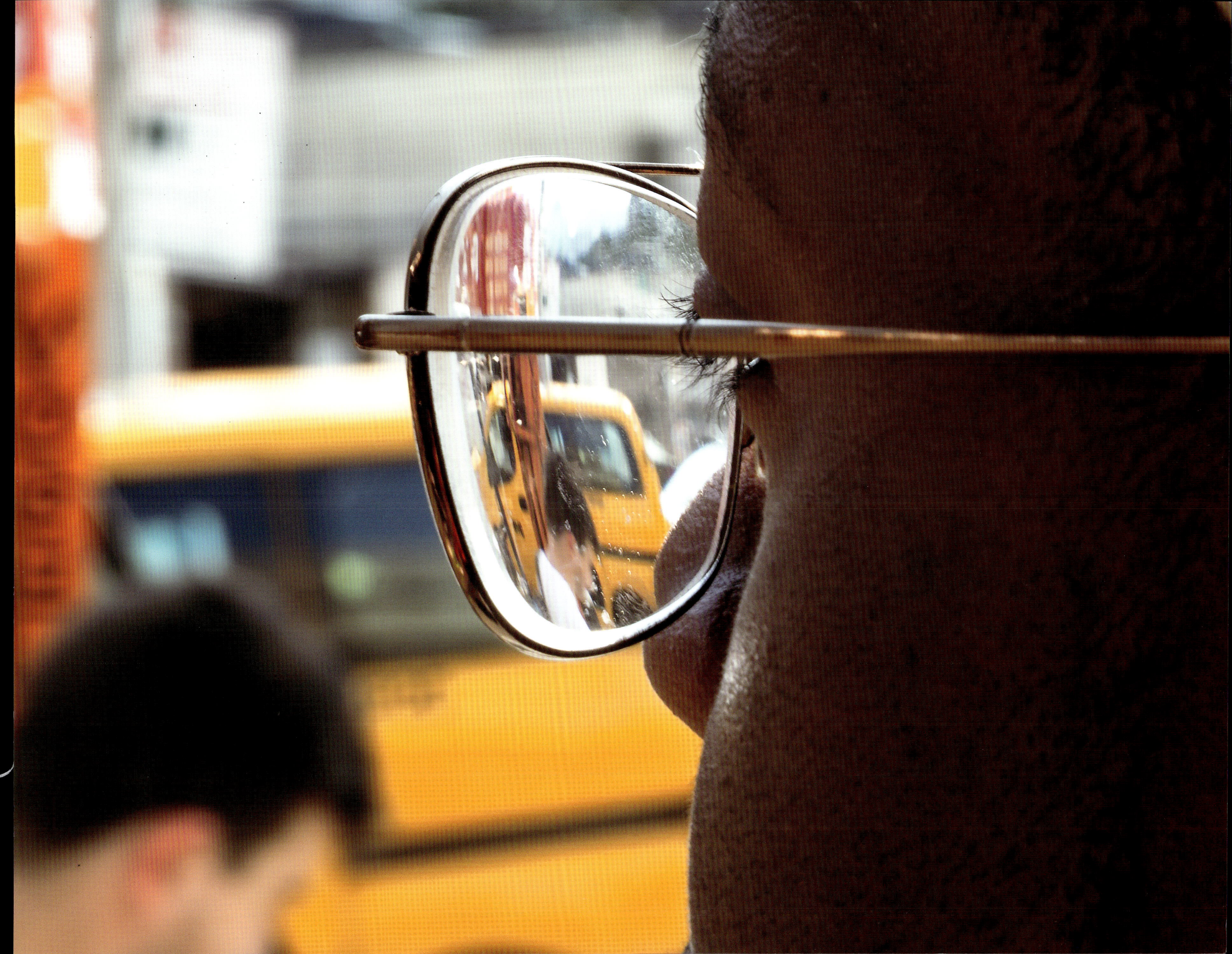

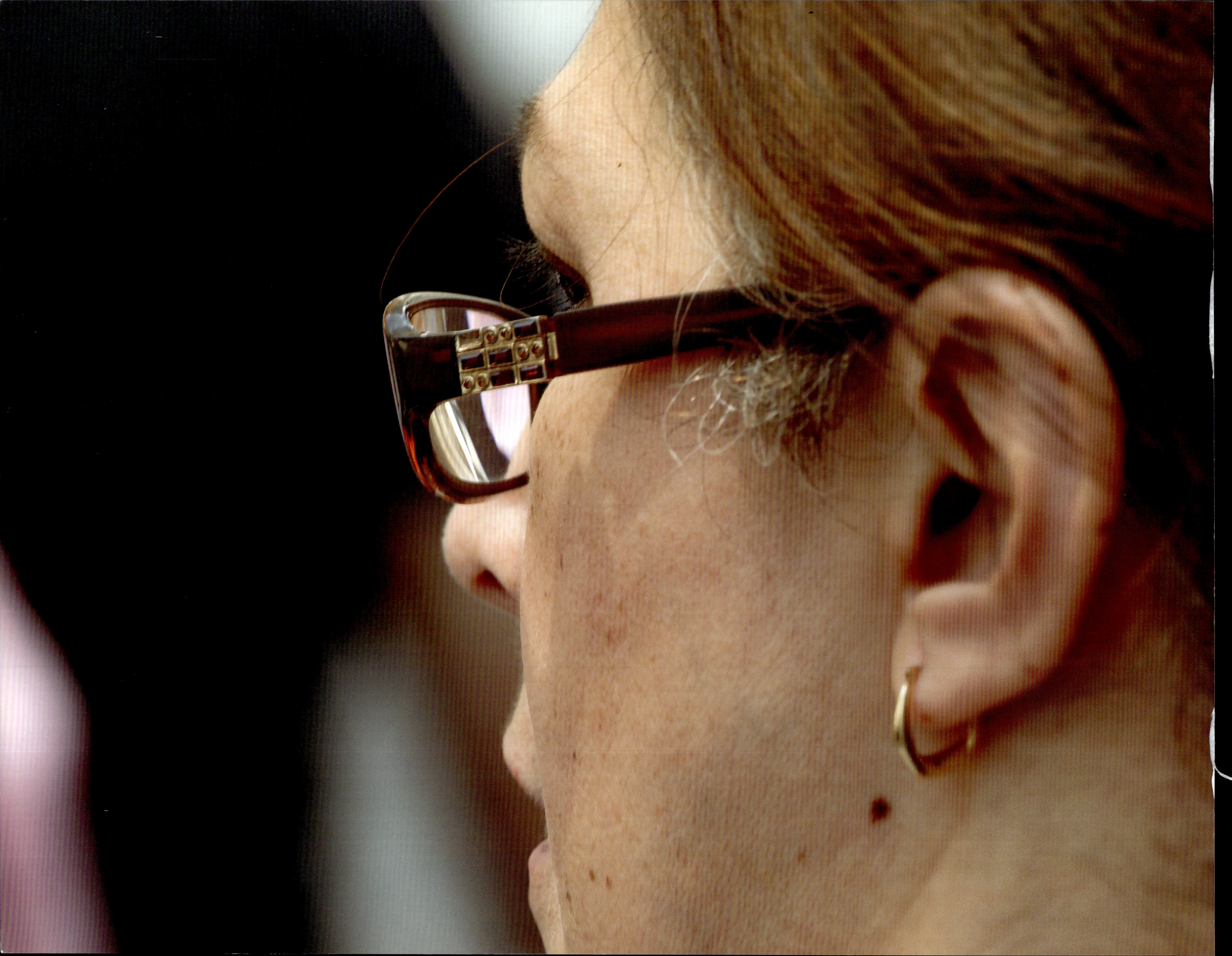

NEIL GOLDBERG: OTHER PEOPLE'S PRESCRIPTIONS

Designed by Tod Lippy

Esopus Books
The Esopus Foundation Ltd.
41 Schermerhorn Street, #143
Brooklyn, New York 11201

ISBN 978-0-9899117-6-4

Distributed by D.A.P. / Distributed Art Publishers, Inc.
75 Broad Street, New York, NY 10004
ARTBOOK.com

Edition of 500
Printed in Canada

Acknowledgments:

Neil Goldberg is pleased to thank the following individuals and institutions (listed alphabetically) for making this publication possible: Bernhard Blythe, Jennifer Callahan, Cristin Tierney Gallery, The Esopus Foundation Ltd., Jeff Hiller, Bridget Leslie, Tod Lippy, Louis Menand, Ria Roberts, Siena Art Institute, Maddy Sinnock, and Charlie Theobald for his invaluable assistance with the "Other People's Prescriptions" series.

Tod Lippy is pleased to thank the following individuals (listed alphabetically) for making this publication possible: Georgia Cool, Neil Goldberg, David Hariton, Keriann Kohler, George Kondogianis, Louis Menand, and Chris Young.